Neurotrauma

Treatment, Rehabilitation, and Related Issues

No. 3

Neurotrauma

Treatment, Rehabilitation, and Related Issues

No. 3

Edited by

Michael E. Miner, *M.D., Ph.D.*

Professor and Director
Division of Neurosurgery
Department of Surgery
University of Texas Medical School at Houston
Houston, Texas

Karen A. Wagner, *Ph.D.*

Assistant Professor
Department of Rehabilitation
Baylor College of Medicine
Houston, Texas

with 33 contributing authors

Butterworths
Boston London Singapore Sydney Toronto Wellington

Library of Congress Cataloging-in-Publication Data

(Revised for Volume 3)

Neurotrauma: Treatment, rehabilitation, and related issues

   Proceedings of the Third Houston Conference on Neurotrauma, held in February 1987.
   Includes bibliographies and index.
   1. Head—Wounds and injuries—Congresses.
2. Brain—Wounds and injuries—Complications and sequelae—Congresses. 3. Head—Wounds and injuries—Patients—Rehabilitation—Congresses. I. Miner, Michael E. II. Wagner, Karen A. III. Houston Conference on Neurotrauma (3rd : 1987) [DNLM: 1. Evoked Potentials—congresses. 2. Head Injuries—rehabilitation—congresses. 3. Head Injuries—therapy—congresses. WE 706 N494 1987]
RD521.N48 1986   617'.48044   86–953
ISBN 0–409–95167–6 (v. 1)
ISBN 0–409–90022–2 (v. 2)
ISBN 0–409–90134–2 (v. 3)

A CIP catalog record for this book is available from the British Library.

Butterworths
80 Montvale Avenue
Stoneham, MA 02180

10 9 8 7 6 5 4 3 2 1

Printed in the United States of America

Contents

Contributing Authors

Steven J. Allen, M.D.
Associate Professor of Anesthesiology, University of Texas Medical School, Houston, Houston, Texas

David C. Anderson, M.D.
Assistant Chief, Department of Neurology, Hennepin County Medical Center, and Associate Professor of Neurology, University of Minnesota, Minneapolis, Minnesota

Brian T. Andrews, M.D.
Department of Neurosurgery, University of California, San Francisco, San Francisco, California

Alan D. Baddeley, Ph.D.
Director, Medical Research Council, Applied Psychology Unit, Cambridge University, Cambridge, England

Juan Cabrera, M.D.
Research Coordinator, Division of Neurosurgery, Department of Surgery, University of Texas Medical School, Houston, Houston, Texas

Janet Cockburn
Psychology Research Worker, Department of Psychology, Rivermead Rehabilitation Centre, Oxford, England

Howard M. Eisenberg, M.D.
Professor and Chief, Department of Surgery, Division of Neurosurgery, University of Texas Medical School, Galveston, Galveston, Texas

Linda Ewing-Cobbs, Ph.D.
Assistant Professor of Psychiatry and Behavioral Sciences, University of Texas Medical School, Houston, Houston, Texas

Jack M. Fletcher, Ph.D.
Associate Professor of Psychology, University of Houston, Houston, Texas

Stephen A. Fletcher, D.O.
Division of Neurosurgery, Department of Surgery, University of Texas Medical School, Houston, Houston, Texas

Sandra E. Ford, R.N.
Research Coordinator, Division of Neurosurgery, Hennepin County Medical Center, Minneapolis, Minnesota

Don Marshall Gash, Ph.D.
Professor of Neurobiology and Anatomy, University of Rochester Medical Center, Rochester, New York

Rolf Habersang, M.D.
Department of Pediatrics, Texas Tech Health Science Center, Amarillo, Texas

James W. Hall III, Ph.D.
Associate Professor and Director of Audiology, Division of Hearing and Speech Sciences, Department of Otolaryngology, Vanderbilt University Medical Center, Nashville, Tennessee

Robin P. Humphreys, M.D., F.R.C.S.C., F.A.C.S.
Associate Surgeon-in-Chief, Hospital for Sick Children, and Associate Professor, Department of Surgery and Anatomy, University of Toronto, Toronto, Canada

Bryan Jennett, M.D., F.R.C.S.
Professor of Neurosurgery, Institute of Neurological Sciences, Southern General Hospital, and Dean of Medicine, University of Glasgow, Glasgow, Scotland

Mark V. Johnston, Ph.D.
Senior Research Analyst, New Medico Head Injury System, Northampton, Massachusetts

Paul Kaufmann, Ph.D.
Research Associate in Neurosurgery, Department of Surgery, University of Texas Medical School, Houston, Houston, Texas

Dennis R. Kopaniky, M.D., Ph.D.
Assistant Professor of Neurosurgery, Department of Surgery, University of Texas Medical School, Houston, Houston, Texas

Madan V. Kulkarni, M.D.
Associate Professor of Radiology, Department of Radiology, University of Texas Medical School, Houston, Houston, Texas

Harvey S. Levin, M.D.
Professor of Surgery, Division of Neurosurgery, University of Texas, Medical Branch at Galveston, Galveston, Texas

Robert MacMillan, B.A.
Data Manager, Department of Neurosurgery, Institute of Neurosurgical Sciences, Southern General Hospital, Glasgow, Scotland

Michael E. Miner, M.D., Ph.D.
Professor and Director of Neurosurgery, Department of Surgery, University of Texas Medical School, Houston, Houston, Texas

Golden Pan, M.D.
Department of Radiology, University of Texas Medical School, Houston, Houston, Texas

Lawrence H. Pitts, M.D.
Associate Professor of Neurosurgery, University of California, San Francisco, and Chief, Department of Neurosurgery, San Francisco General Hospital, San Francisco, California

Robert W. Rand, Ph.D., J.D., M.D.
Professor of Neurological Surgery, Department of Surgery/Neurosurgery, University of California, Los Angeles, Los Angeles, California

Gaylan L. Rockswold, M.D., Ph.D.
Chief, Division of Neurosurgery, Hennepin County Medical Center, and Associate Professor, Department of Neurosurgery, University of Minnesota, Minneapolis, Minnesota

Mitchell Rosenthal, Ph.D.
Director, Psychological Medicine, Marianjoy Rehabilitation Center, Wheaton, Illinois, and Associate Professor of Psychology and Physical Medicine and Rehabilitation, Rush Medical College, Chicago, Illinois

Denise A. Tucker, M.C.D.
Department of Otolaryn-Head and Neck Surgery, Division of Audiology, University of Virginia, Charlottesville, Virginia

Harry C. White, M.D.
Department of Neurobiology and Anatomy, University of Rochester Medical Center, Rochester, New York

L. James Willmore, M.D.
Department of Neurology, University of Texas Medical School, Houston, Houston, Texas

Barbara A. Wilson, Ph.D.
Department of Rehabilitation, Southampton General Hospital, Southampton, England

Joel W. Yeakley, M.D.
Associate Professor, Chief of Neuroradiology, Department of Radiology, University of Texas Medical School, Houston, Texas

Preface

This volume was stimulated by the Third Houston Conference on Neurotrauma, whose history is to bring together specialists with expertise in the management of traumatically brain-injured individuals. The conference forum enables the varied participants to present, discuss, and critique issues relevant from the time of injury through the lifetime recovery process. A special section of this conference, and of this volume, concerns the treatment of traumatic brain injury in children. Acute technological needs, as well as rehabilitation, and long-term needs and strategies, continue to be discussed with increased fervor as the number of brain-injured survivors increases and the allocation of scarce resources becomes more ethically challenging.

We are indebted to Anne Brown and Dr. Daniel Morrison of the Medical Center Del Oro Hospital; to Dr. Catherine Bontke, Marjorie Gordon, and Dr. Don Lehmkuhl of The Institute for Rehabilitation and Research; and to Lou Esposito and Gloria Horner of The University of Texas Medical School, Houston; for their help in planning the conference and their support in the preparation of this book.

M.E.M.
K.A.W.

Neurotrauma

Treatment, Rehabilitation, and Related Issues

No. 3

Part I
The Role of Technology and Assessment of Brain Injury

Michael E. Miner

The gold standard of medical decision making with regard to brain injury has been the neurologic examination. This has truly stood the test of time. However, we do have technology that can explore subclinical abnormalities, expand clinical observations, and increase objectivity in patient management. Bryan Jennett is commonly cast in the role of exposing the abuses of technology. Here, however, he categorizes technology into tools that provide data and tools that can be used in interventions to treat abnormalities. He reminds us that technology must be paid for, whether through improvement in existing care or through more efficient use of resources. Technologies that improve patient care must be distinguished from those that merely satisfy the curiosity of the physician. Professor Jennett acknowledges that new technologies must be tested, but tested in such a way that the value of the technology can be determined. Technology assessment must be done under conditions that can provide real answers to such compelling questions as: "Is this a technology that improves patient outcome?" and "What is the price?" Test results must not consist merely of a series of anecdotal experiences but statistically valid answers.

Recently, clinical data have seemed to take a secondary position to technology. If the CT scan says the lesion is in the frontal lobe but the clinical examination says the parietal lobe, where does the surgeon make the scalp incision? The answer is obvious. Clinicians have become very cautious about their observations and feel that they must substantiate them with other data. However, clinical data are the backbone of medicine. Brian Andrews and Lawrence Pitts review this problem with regard to emergency treatment of brain injury. They eloquently recount their experience with intracranial surgery based upon clinical findings alone. They report on a subset of brain-injured patients they thought would benefit from exploratory surgery and in whom delay for diagnostic tests was not warranted. These dying patients clearly benefited from rapid surgery. Such "woodpecker surgery," involving multiple burr holes, has gone out of vogue since CT has become so readily available. However, there is still a delay whenever diagnostic tests are obtained, and that delay must be carefully weighed against both the dynamics of the pathologic process involved and the severity of the injury. Andrews and Pitts find that there is indeed a place for surgery based only on the clinical examination. This is a refreshing observation in our highly technologic society.

"Flying blind" is not a reasonable course, whether that blindness is to data, time, or pathophysiology. Data derived from machines must be interpreted just as data derived from clinical examination of patients. Judgment implies an understanding of the options available and a reasonable grasp of the benefits and risks of a series of decisions. Technology that aids in this process is always needed, but new technologies should not be assumed to be of value before they are tested.

Chapter 1

Neural Transplants: Potential Applications for Treating Brain Damage

Harry C. White
Don Marshall Gash

Despite the common clinical observation of significant, though frequently incomplete, recovery of function following brain injury in humans (e.g., traumatic brain injury, stroke, or ablative neurosurgical procedures), the search for the neurobiological substrates of clinical recovery patterns remains problematic. Intensive therapy is typically directed toward the resolution of secondary pathophysiology (e.g., ischemia, edema, hemorrhage, increased intracranial pressure, or impaired metabolic regulation). In many clinical settings the rehabilitation of individuals with central nervous system (CNS) injury is underutilized and underexplored. In the absence of a generally agreed upon theoretical framework, this failure to apply available empirical strategies to optimize function is partially explained by the apparent enigma of recovery of function. Is it possible that what works in practice cannot work in theory?

Classical theories, such as redundancy or equipotentiation (the sparing of uninjured neural pathways normally not contributing to a task), vicariation or functional reorganization (the mediation of recovery through alternative pathways), and release from diaschisis (functional depression of structures remote from, but connected to, the site of injury), are extremely difficult to subject to meaningful hypothesis testing. Patrick Wall has termed these theories "mystical" solutions to the problem of recovery, that is names that imply understanding but only describe a process they pretend to explain[1].

Alternatively, attempts have been made to operationalize clinical recovery as either (1) adaptive recovery, that is, behavioral compensation for an impairment, using problem-solving strategies centered on spared abilities, or (2) neurologic recovery, regaining neural control over lost function. Although superficially attractive, this dichotomization of recovery may cloud as much as it enlightens. In so-called adaptive recovery the necessary requirement for intact learning will be dependent on neural substrates, which themselves require further explanation. Conversely, neural recovery may require a substituted behavioral pattern (i.e., a learned adaptive strategy) for the achievement of some functional goal. Both adaptive and neural modes of recovery are likely to be experience-dependent for optimization of function and, therefore, potentially responsive to rehabilitation.

Ramón y Cajal contended early in this century that the brain possessed a tendency toward natural regeneration frustrated not by "essential, fatal, and unchangeable conditions," but "by two negative conditions: (1) the lack of substances able to sustain and invigorate the indolent and scanty growth of the sprouts, and (2) the absence in the paths or systems of interrupted nerve fibers of catalytic agents capable of attracting and directing the axonic current to its destination" [2]. For most of the 20th Century, however, discussion of any inherent reparative capacity in the adult mammalian CNS was tabled by the dominant conceptualization of the brain as a fixed, immutable structure without significant capacity for structural or functional reorganization.

Experimental work by Liu and Chambers [3] on the compensatory sprouting of spared dorsal root fibers into the spinal cord, and by Goodman and Horel [4] showing axonal sprouting of optic tract projections after ablation of the occipital cortex, set the stage for a major paradigmatic shift [5]. The publication of Geoffrey Raisman's 1969 report, providing ultrastructural evidence of synaptic modification after partial deafferentation of the septal nucleus in the adult rat [6], heralded the "construction" of neuronal plasticity as a "fact" [7].

With the "thought style" [8] of neuronal plasticity having begun to supplant the earlier emphasis on the rigidity of CNS structures, conditions were favorable for the reconsideration of grafting of neural tissue into the CNS of mammals. Since the turn of the century, attempts at transplantation of mammalian nervous tissue had been sporadic and limited in success [see 9,10 for reviews]. What might be called the modern era of neural transplantation began in the early 1970s: the experimental methodology of Olson et al [11,12], who used the anterior chamber of the eye as a site for transplantation of mammalian CNS tissue; the work of Das and Altman [13,14] on the transplantation of fetal neurons into the cerebelli of neonatal rats; the studies of Björklund and Stenevi and their colleagues [15–17] demonstrating the innervation of implants of peripheral tissue by regenerating CNS axons; and the observations of Lund and Hauschka [18] on the innervation of fetal superior colliculus transplanted into newborn rat visual pathways. Perhaps the most significant studies among these pioneering experiments were those of Björklund and Stenevi [19,20] demonstrating the feasibility of grafting fetal neuronal tissue into the adult mammalian nervous system.

In the past decade transplantation methodologies have been applied to a number of model systems of CNS pathology, including lesions of the nigrostriatal dopaminergic system [21–23]; cholinergic deafferentation of the hippocampus [24–26]; frontal lobe lesions [27,28]; damage to the basal forebrain [29,30]; neuroendocrine dysfunction [31–34]; striatal injury [35–38]; and age-associated behavioral impairments [39–42]. In addition to attempts to ameliorate neural dysfunction, neural grafting has also proved useful in the study of the regulation of axonal growth, the ontogeny of synaptic connectivity, and the exploration of the inherent neuronal plasticity of neural systems. A variety of morphological, biochemical, electrophysiological, and behavioral measures have been employed as outcome criteria in these studies.

Four major technical strategies have emerged: (1) solid graft placement into preformed cavities [20]; (2) intraparenchymal injection of cellular suspensions [43]; (3) graft placement into ventricular cavities [21,44,45]; and (4) the use of peripheral nervous system tissue as a "bridge" for axonal growth [46,47]. The most common source of neural tissue remains embryonal tissue from syngeneic donors, although the use of nonfetal sources (e.g., adrenal medullary autografts [21,48] or differentiated tumor cell lines [49–52]) is currently under evaluation in a number of laboratories.

The functional effects of neural grafts have generally been accounted for on the basis of one of two hypothesized mechanisms: the formation of synaptic connections to reestablish damaged neural circuits, or the local release of neuroactive substances [see 53 for review]. Björklund and colleagues [54] report that the implantation of a suspension of fetal ventral forebrain neurons following cholinergic deafferentation of the hippocampus in the adult rat results in a partial functional restoration of behavioral impairment, and is also associated with the formation of cholinergic synapses, as established by electron microscopic immunocytochemistry for choline acetyltransferase (ultrastructural evidence of cholinergic synapses in this model system has also been reported by Anderson et al. [55]) and electrophysiological evidence of graft innervation of the host [23,56,57]. Correlation of morphological, electrophysiological, and behavioral results in the septal-lesioned rat suggests that functional synaptic connectivity between graft and host is a necessary condition for behavioral recovery. Alternatively, experimental designs in which fetal neural tissue or adrenal medulla is implanted into ventricular spaces [21,31,48,58,59] are most easily explained on the basis of the local release of neuroactive substances (e.g., catecholamines or neuropeptides), either into the cerebrospinal fluid bath surrounding the graft or via neurohemal connections with adjacent fenestrated blood vessels.

A small but growing body of data has focused interest on a third possible mechanism for the biological activity of neural grafts, graft-related trophic properties. As discussed in the following paragraphs, it is now highly plausible that the relationship between the neural graft and the host animal includes reciprocal trophic interactions. Host trophic factors may support the survival and growth of neural transplants, whereas neuronotrophic activity originating in the graft may enhance functional recovery in the damaged host. Each element of the relationship, the host system and the implanted graft, potentially contributes to the maintenance of the other.

Nieto-Sampedro, Cotman, and colleagues have documented soluble trophic factor(s), elicited by injury to the host CNS, that resulted in the enhanced survival of neural grafts [60,61]. In vitro measures of neuronotrophic activity demonstrated titers that were induced by injury; peak levels occurred one to two weeks after the lesion and were followed by a gradual decay. Trophic activity was positively correlated with the improved survival of cortical grafts [60]. Extracts of the wound site adsorbed onto Gelfoam® sponge were also effective in vivo. Transplants placed into cortical wound cavities immediately postlesion showed poor survival characteristics. When supplemented by wound extracts, graft survival was improved [61].

Gage and Björklund have argued for a degree of selectivity of injury-induced neurotrophic factors [62]. Increased survival of fetal ventral forebrain neurons implanted into the hippocampus (as measured by graft volume, number of cholinergic neurons, and level of choline acetyltransferase activity) was noted in animals that received fimbria-fornix lesions compared with sham nondenervated controls, but no improvement in animals that received lesions to the retrosplenial cortex. They concluded that the enhancing effects of cholinergic denervation of the hippocampus were independent of a nonspecific, wound-induced agent.

Observations from a number of laboratories support the theoretical supposition of what might be thought of as the complementary phenomenon, functional recovery of the host CNS influenced by graft-related neuronotrophic factors. Aguayo et al [63,64] have pioneered the use of peripheral nerve grafts to study axonal regeneration from central neurons. They have demonstrated that the microenvironment, provided by the nonneuronal elements of peripheral nerve segments transplanted into the CNS, is able to promote and support the elongation of axotomized neurites into the graft. In a somewhat analogous experiment, Kromer et al [65] described the capacity of embryonic hippocampus to serve as a tissue "bridge" in promoting the regeneration of cholinergic fibers originating in the septum and the partial reinnervation of previously denervated hippocampus. Again using the model system of cholinergic deafferentation of the hippocampus following septal lesions, Kromer and Cornbrooks [66] provided evidence on the role of cultured Schwann cells in facilitating the regeneration of acetylcholinesterase-positive fibers.

Recently, several laboratories have reported on the ability of neural transplants to protect host neurons from atrophy or death, secondary to either axotomy or excitatory amino acids. Bregman and Reier have shown that the transplantation of embryonic spinal cord into the lesioned spinal cords of newborn rats was able to spare rubrospinal perikarya from the anticipated retrograde degeneration after axotomy [67]. In a complex model involving sequential bilateral kainic acid lesions to the striatum, Tulipan et al have reported a substantial reduction in mortality and the sparing of the contralateral striatum, when the first lesion is followed by the ipsilateral implantation of neural tissue [68]. As demonstrated by Sofroniew et al, the neocortical implantation of fetal cortex grafts seems to exert a protective influence on the atrophy seen in nucleus basalis neurons following kainic acid damage to cortex

[69]. All three experiments are consistent with the existence of a neurotrophic influence by the graft exerted on the host.

Labbe et al have reported a reduction in learning impairments after bilateral frontal cortex lesions followed by the transplantation of fetal cortex [27]. Despite their identification of neural connections between the host and implant after two to five months of survival, the time course of improvement in the performance of the spatial alternation task (four days) seemed too rapid to be explained on the basis of reestablished neural pathways; this raises the possibility that the observed recovery was mediated by an alternative mechanism, such as neurotrophic factors. Using a similar experimental design, Kesslak et al have demonstrated that the transplantation of cultured astrocytes or Gelfoam previously adsorbed on the lesion site of another animal, but not cell-free extracts of the wound Gelfoam, resulted in a significant improvement in the learning impairment [28]. Because of the requirement for a cellular preparation, they speculated on the possible role of glia in stabilizing the neuronal environment, in addition to the possible elaboration of trophic substances.

Discussion of possible clinical applications for neural grafting has usually been limited to a consideration of interventive strategies in various neurodegenerative diseases (e.g., Alzheimer's, Parkinson's, or Huntington's). Because the affected neuronal populations in these disease entities are known to some extent, degenerative diseases of the CNS are particularly attractive candidates for potential clinical trials. Although the neuropathology of each undoubtedly involves more than the deficiency of a single neurotransmitter, the concept of replacing dead or dysfunctional neurons with a neurotransmitter-specific cell population has seemed feasible. Indeed, clinical trials of adrenal medullary autografts for the treatment of refractory Parkinsonism are currently under way at three sites: the Karolinska Institute in Stockholm [70], the Universidad Nacional Autónoma de México in Mexico City [71], and the Capital Institute of Medicine in Beijing (Dr. Shou-Shu Jiao, personal communication, 1987). In anticipation of possible clinical trials involving the use of fetal human neural tissue, several laboratories have begun to investigate the efficacy of human fetal substantia nigra grafted into animal models of Parkinson's disease [72,73]. Because of the social, ethical, and legal issues raised by the use of human fetal neural tissue in clinical trials, other laboratories, including our own, are testing alternative nonfetal sources for neural grafts that might be employed clinically. These include differentiated amitotic tumor cell lines [49–52] and paraneural tissue [59,74].

In contrast to the intense research effort given to the potential application of grafts for the treatment of neurodegenerative diseases, little effort has been directed toward the use of neural transplants to treat closed head injury. Because of the diffuse nature of neural pathology that has been described in closed head injury [75,76], the transplantation strategies proposed for treating neurodegenerative diseases, for the most part focused on specific neural systems, would appear inappropriate.

Three proposed modes of action of neural grafts were discussed earlier: local production of neuroactive substances, restoration of neuronal connectivity, and promotion of host neural plasticity. The first, use of implanted neural tissue as a chemical generator (e.g., dopamine in Parkinson's disease), appears to have limited rationale in our current understanding of recovery of function following brain injury.

The second, which might be metaphorically thought of as functional rewiring of neuronal circuitry, seems most germane in a consideration of focal brain damage (e.g., frontal lobe injury). Although there is evidence for the formation of neural connections between graft and host in transplantation after frontal lobe ablation [27], the morphologic organization of neocortical grafts appears abnormal [77]. As discussed earlier, Cotman's laboratory has recently reported on the capacity of purified astrocytes to facilitate functional recovery after frontal cortex ablation [28]. In addition, Stein et al [78] have shown a partial restoration of visual deficits after bilateral occipital cortex damage with embryonic frontal cortical grafts, but not with transplants of embryonic occipital cortex. Experiments such as these lend credence to the hypothesis that neural grafting after neocortical ablations may be mediated by the production of neurotrophic factors, rather than the reestablishment of neural connections between host and graft. Whatever the mechanism of action, it is certainly plausible that neural grafting may some day play a role in the treatment of circumscribed focal injuries to the CNS.

Given the prevalence of diffuse neural injury seen after brain trauma, the third mode of function, an enhancement of the inherent regenerative capacity of the host, may be particularly relevant. A number of laboratories have provided data in support of the hypothesis that grafts may function either by sparing host neural tissue from delayed injury (e.g., retrograde degeneration after axonal injury or neuronal protection from damage mediated by excitotoxins) or by providing substrate-bound or soluble neurotrophic factors that influence axonal regeneration or collateral sprouting [28,45,46,66–69,79].

The mechanisms underlying these observations of structural and behavioral amelioration of injury are currently unknown. Speculation includes glial stabilization of the neural microenvironment [28]; neurotrophic ("growth") factors supporting neuronal survival, axonal elongation, and reactive synaptogenesis; and trophic influences determining directionality of growth. As studies of this kind continue to delineate basic principles of neuronal plasticity and recovery of function, the optimal strategy may prove to be one of using defined chemical factors (e.g., the administration of neurotrophic factors) to promote inherent recovery mechanisms without resorting to the use of neural grafts.

We have entered an era in which significant progress is being made in the field of neuronal plasticity. Although long an area of pragmatic importance, research in the neurobiological substrates of recovery of function has become an area of great theoretical importance as well. We are optimistic that individuals with traumatic brain injury will share the fruits of current work in the area of neural transplantation. It remains to be seen whether the applications are direct and include transplantation therapy, or are the more indirect result of an increased understanding of the mechanisms of regeneration.

REFERENCES

1. Wall PD. Mechanisms of plasticity of connection following damage in adult mammalian nervous systems. In: Bach-y-Rita, ed. Recovery of function: theoretical considerations for brain injury rehabilitation. Baltimore: University Park Press, 1980;91–105.
2. Ramón y Cajal S. Degeneration and regeneration of the nervous system (May RM, trans.). London:Oxford University Press, 1928.
3. Liu C-N, Chambers WW. Intraspinal sprouting of dorsal root axons. Arch Neurol Psychiatr 1958;79:46–61.
4. Goodman DC, Horel JA. Sprouting of optic tract projections in the brain stem of the rat. J Comp Neurol 1964;127:71–88.
5. Kuhn TS. The structure of scientific revolutions, 2nd ed. Chicago: University of Chicago, 1970
6. Raisman G. Neuronal plasticity in the septal nuclei of the adult rat. Brain Res 1969;14:25–48.
7. Latour B, Woolgar S. Laboratory life: the construction of scientific facts, 2nd ed. Princeton, NJ: Princeton University, 1986.
8. Fleck L. Genesis and development of a scientific fact. In: Tress TJ, Merton RK, eds; Brady F, Tress TJ, trans. Chicago: University of Chicago, 1979.
9. Gash DM. Neural transplants in mammals: a historical overview. In: Sladek JR Jr, Gash DM, eds. Neural transplants: development and function. New York: Plenum Press, 1984;1:1–12.
10. Björklund A, Stenevi U. Intracerebral neural grafting: a historical perspective. In: Björklund A, Stenevi U, eds. Neural grafting in the mammalian CNS. Amsterdam: Elsevier 1985;1:3–14.
11. Olson L, Malmfors T. Growth characteristics of adrenergic nerves in the adult rat. Fluorescence histochemical and 3H-noradrenaline uptake studies using tissue transplantation to the anterior chamber of the eye. Acta Physiol Scand (Suppl) 1970;348:1–112.
12. Hoffer BJ, Seiger Å, Ljungberg T, Olson L. Electrophysiological and cytological studies of brain homografts in the anterior chamber of the eye. Maturation of cerebellar cortex in oculo. Brain Res 1974;79:165–84.
13. Das GD, Altman J. Transplanted precursors of nerve cells: their fate in the cerebellums of young rats. Science 1971;173:637-38.
14. Das GD, Altman J. Studies on the transplantation of developing nervous tissue in the mammalian brain. I. Transplantation of cerebellar slabs into the cerebellum of neonate brains. Brain Res 1972;38:233–49.
15. Björklund A, Stenevi U. Growth of central catecholamine neurons into smooth muscle grafts in the rat mesencephalon. Brain Res 1971;31:1–20.
16. Bjerre B, Björklund A, Stenevi U. Stimulation of growth of new axonal sprouts from lesioned monoamine neurons in adult rat brain by nerve growth factor. Brain Res 1973;60:161–76.
17. Svendgarrd N-Aa, Björklund A, Stenevi U. Regeneration of central cholinergic neurons in the adult rat brain. Brain Res 1976;102:1–22.

18. Lund RD, Hauschka SD. Transplanted neural tissue develops connections with host rat brain. Science 1976;193:582–84.
19. Björklund A, Stenevi U. Growth of transplanted monoaminergic neurones into the adult hippocampus along the perforant path. Nature (London) 1976;262:787–90.
20. Stenevi U, Björklund A, Svendgaard N-Aa. Transplantation of central and peripheral monoamine neurons to the adult rat brain: techniques and conditions for survival. Brain Res 1976;114:1–20.
21. Perlow MJ, Freed WJ, Hoffer BJ, Seiger Å, Olson L, Wyatt RJ. Brain grafts reduce motor abnormalities produced by destruction of nigrostriatal dopamine system. Science 1979;204:643–47.
22. Björklund A, Dunnett SB, Stenevi U, Lewis ME, Iversen SD. Reinnervation of the denervated striatum by substantia nigra transplants: functional consequences as revealed by pharmacological and sensorimotor testing. Brain Res 1980;199:307–33.
23. Redmond DE, Sladek JR Jr, Roth RH, Collier TJ, Elsworth JD, Deutch AY, Haber S. Fetal neuronal grafts in monkeys given methylphenyltetrahydropyridine. Lancet 1986;1:1125–27.
24. Björklund A, Stenevi U. Reformation of the severed septohippocampal cholinergic pathway in the adult rat by transplanted septal neurones. Cell Tissue Res 1977;185:289–302.
25. Dunnett SB, Low WC, Iversen SD, Stenevi U, Björklund A. Septal transplants restore maze learning in rats with fimbria-fornix lesions. Brain Res 1982;251:335–48.
26. Low WC, Lewis PR, Bunch ST, Dunnett SB, Thomas SR, Iversen SD, Björklund A, Stenevi U. Functional recovery following transplantation of embryonic septal nuclei into adult rats with septohippocampal lesions. Nature (London) 1982;300:260-62.
27. Labbe R, Firl A Jr, Mufson EJ, Stein DG. Fetal brain transplants: reduction of cognitive deficits in rats with frontal cortex lesions. Science 1983;221:470–72.
28. Kesslak JP, Nieto-Sampedro M, Globus J, Cotman CW. Transplants of purified astrocytes promote behavioral recovery after frontal cortex ablation. Exp Neurol 1986;92:377–90.
29. Dunnett SB, Toniolo G, Fine A, Ryan CN, Björklund A, Iversen SD. Transplantation of embryonic ventral forebrain neurons to the neocortex of rats with lesions of nucleus basalis magnocellularis. II. Sensorimotor and learning impairments. Neuroscience 1985:16:787–95.
30. Fine A, Dunnett SB, Björklund A, Clarke D, Iversen SD. Transplantation of embryonic ventral forebrain neurons to the neocortex of rats with lesions of nucleus basalis magnocellularis. I. Biochemical and anatomical observations. Neuroscience 1985;16:769–86.
31. Gash DM, Sladek JR Jr, Sladek CD. Functional development of grafted vasopressin neurons. Science 1980;210:1367–69.
32. Krieger DT, Perlow MJ, Gibson MJ, Dames TF, Zimmerman EA, Ferin M, Charlton HM. Brain grafts reverse hypogonadism of gonadotropin-releasing hormone deficiency. Nature (London) 1982;298:468–71.
33. Arendash GW, Leung PCK. Alleviation of estrogen-induced hyperprolactinemia through intracerebral transplantation of hypothalamic tissue containing dopaminergic neurons. Neuroendocrinology 1986;43:359–67.

34. Marciano FF, Gash DM. Structural and functional relationships of grafted vasopressin neurons. Brain Res 1986;370:338–42.
35. Deckel AW, Robinson RG, Coyle JT, Sanberg PR. Reversal of locomotor abnormalities in the kainic acid model of Huntington's disease by day 18 fetal striatal implants. Eur J Pharmacol 1983;93:287-88.
36. Isacson O, Brundin P, Kelly P, Gage FH, Björklund A. Functional neuronal replacement by grafted neurons in the ibotenic acid-lesioned striatum. Nature (London) 1984;311:458–60.
37. Isacson O, Dunnett SB, Björklund A. Graft-induced behavioral recovery in an animal model of Huntington's disease. Proc Natl Acad Sci 1986;83:2728–32.
38. Deckel AW, Moran TH, Coyle JT, Sanberg PR, Robinson RG. Anatomical predictors of behavioral recovery following fetal striatal transplants. Brain Res 1986;365:249–58.
39. Gage FH, Dunnett SB, Stenevi U, Björklund A. Aged rats: recovery of motor impairments by intrastriatal nigral grafts. Science 1983;221:966–69.
40. Gage FH, Björklund A, Stenevi U, Dunnett SB, Kelly PAT. Intrahippocampal septal grafts ameliorate learning impairments in aged rats. Science 1984;225:533–36.
41. Collier TJ, Gash DM, Bruemmer V, Sladek JR Jr. Impaired regulation of arousal in old age and the consequences for learning and memory: replacement of brain norepinephrine via neuron transplants improves memory performance in aged F344 rats. In: Davis BB, Wood WG, eds. Homeostatic function and aging. New York: Raven Press, 1985;95–110.
42. Gage FH, Björklund A. Cholinergic septal grafts into the hippocampal formation improve spatial learning and memory in aged rats by an atropine-sensitive mechanism. J Neurosci 1986;6:2837–47.
43. Björklund A, Schmidt RH, Stenevi U. Functional reinnervation of the neostriatum in the adult rat by use of intraparenchymal grafting of dissociated cell suspensions from the substantia nigra. Cell Tissue Res 1980;212:39–45.
44. Rosenstein JM, Brightman MW. Intact cerebral ventricle as a site for tissue transplantation. Nature (London) 1978;276:83–85.
45. Gash DM, Sladek JR Jr. Vasopressin neurons grafted into Brattleboro rats: viability and activity. Peptides 1980;1:11–14.
46. Aguayo AJ, Björklund A, Stenevi U, Carlstedt T. Fetal mesencephalic neurons survive and extend long axons across PNS grafts inserted into the adult rat striatum. Neurosci Lett 1984;45:53–58.
47. Gage FH, Stenevi U, Carlstedt T, Foster G, Björklund A, Aguayo AJ. Anatomical and functional consequences of grafting mesencephalic neurons into a peripheral nerve "bridge" connected to the denervated striatum. Exp Brain Res 1985;60:584–89.
48. Sagen J, Pappas GD, Pollard HB. Analgesia induced by isolated bovine chromaffin cells implanted in rat spinal cord. Proc Natl Acad Sci 1986;83:7522–26.
49. Gash DM, Notter MFD, Dick LB, Kraus AL, Okawara SH, Wechkin SW, Joynt RJ. Cholinergic neurons transplanted into the neocortex and hippocampus of primates: studies on African Green monkeys. In: Björklund A, Stenevi U, eds. Neural grafting in the mammalian CNS. Amsterdam: Elsevier, 1985;51:595–603.
50. Gash DM, Notter MFD, Okawara SH, Kraus LA, Joynt RJ. Amitotic neuroblastoma cells used for neural implants in monkeys. Science 1986;233:1420–22.

51. Freed WJ, Patel-Vaidya U, Geller, HM. Properties of PC12 pheochromocytoma cells transplanted to the adult rat brain. Exp Brain Res 1986;63:557–66.
52. Kordower JH, Notter MFD, Gash DM. Neuroblastoma cells and neural transplantation: a neuroanatomical and behavioral analysis. Brain Res 1987;417:85–98.
53. Björklund A, Stenevi U. Intracerebral neural implants: neuronal replacement and reconstruction of damaged circuitries. Annu Rev Neurosci 1984;7:279–308.
54. Clarke DJ, Gage FH, Björklund A. Formation of cholinergic synapses by intrahippocampal septal grafts as revealed by choline acetyltransferase immunocytochemistry. Brain Res 1986;369:151–62.
55. Anderson KJ, Gibbs RB, Salvaterra PM, Cotman CW. Ultrastructural characterization of identified cholinergic neurons transplanted to the hippocampal formation of the rat. J Comp Neurol 1986;249:279–92.
56. Segal M, Björklund A, Gage FH. Transplanted septal neurons make viable cholinergic synapses with a host hippocampus. Brain Res 1985;336:302–7.
57. Buzsáki G, Gage FH, Czopf J, Björklund A. Restoration of rhythmic slow activity (theta) in the subcortically denervated hippocampus by fetal CNS transplants. Brain Res 1987;400:334–47.
58. Freed WJ, Perlow MJ, Karoum F, Seiger Å, Olson L, Hoffer BJ, Wyatt RJ. Restoration of dopaminergic function by grafting of fetal rat substantia nigra to the caudate nucleus: long-term behavioral, biochemical, and histochemical studies. Ann Neurol 1980;8:510–19.
59. Freed WJ, Morihisa JM, Spoor E, Hoffer BJ, Olson L, Seiger Å, Wyatt RJ. Transplanted adrenal chromaffin cells in rat brain reduce lesion-induced rotational behavior. Nature (London) 1981;292:351–52.
60. Nieto-Sampedro M, Manthorpe M, Barbin G, Varon S, Cotman CW. Injury-induced neuronotrophic activity in adult rat brain: correlation with survival of delayed implants in the wound cavity. J Neurosci 1983;3:2219–29.
61. Nieto-Sampedro M, Whittemore SR, Needels DL, Larson J, Cotman CW. The survival of brain transplants is enhanced by extracts from injured brain. Proc Natl Acad Sci 1984;81:6250–54.
62. Gage FH, Björklund A. Enhanced graft survival in the hippocampus following selective denervation. Neuroscience 1986;17:89–98.
63. Richardson PM, McGuinness UM, Aguayo AJ. Axons from CNS neurons regenerate into PNS grafts. Nature (London) 1980;284:264–265.
64. David S, Aguayo AJ. Axonal elongation into PNS "bridges" after CNS injury in adult rats. Science 1981;214:931–33.
65. Kromer LF, Björklund A, Stenevi U. Regeneration of the septohippocampal pathways in adult rats is promoted by utilizing embryonic hippocampal implants as bridges. Brain Res 1981;210:173–200.
66. Kromer LF, Cornbrooks CJ. Transplants of Schwann cell cultures promote axonal regeneration in the adult mammalian brain. Proc Natl Acad Sci 1985;82:6330–34.
67. Bregman BS, Reier PJ. Neural tissue transplants rescue axotomized rubrospinal cells from retrograde death. J Comp Neurol 1986;244:86–95.
68. Tulipan M, Huang S, Whetsell WO, Allen GS. Neonatal striatal grafts prevent lethal syndrome produced by bilateral intrastriatal injection of kainic acid. Brain Res 1986;377:163–77.
69. Sofroniew MV, Isacson O, Björklund A. Cortical grafts prevent atrophy of cholinergic basal nucleus neurons induced by excitotoxic cortical damage. Brain Res 1986;378:409–16.

70. Backlund E-O, Granberg P-O, Hamberger B, Knuttson E, Mårtensson A, Sedvall G, Seiger Å, Olson L. Transplantation of adrenal medullary tissue to the striatum in parkinsonism: first clinical trials. J Neurosurg 1985;62:169–73.
71. Madrazo I, Drucker-Colín R, Díaz V, Martínez-Mata J, Torres C, Becerril JJ. Open microsurgical autograft of adrenal medulla to the right caudate nucleus in two patients with intractable Parkinson's disease. N Engl J Med 1987;316:831–34.
72. Strömberg I, Bygdeman M, Goldstein M, Seiger Å, Olson L. Human fetal substantia nigra grafted to the dopamine-denervated striatum of immunosuppressed rats: evidence for functional reinnervation. Neurosci Lett 1986;71:271–76.
73. Brundin P, Nilsson OG, Strecker RE, Lindvall O, Åstedt B, Björklund A. Behavioral effects of human fetal dopamine neurons grafted in a rat model of Parkinson's disease. Exp Brain Res 1986;65:235–40.
74. Bing G, Notter MFD, Hansen J, Gash DM. Comparison of PC12, adrenal medulla, and glomus cell grafts in 6-OHDA lesioned rats. Brain Res Bull 1988;20:399–406.
75. Adams JH, Graham DI, Gennarelli TA. Contemporary neuropathological considerations regarding brain damage in head injury. In: Becker DP, Povlishock JT, eds. Central nervous system trauma status report. Richmond: William Byrd, 1985;4:65–77.
76. Adams JH, Graham DI, Murray LS, Scott G. Diffuse axonal injury due to nonmissile head injury in humans: and analysis of 45 cases. Ann Neurol 1982;12:557–63.
77. Mufson EJ, Labbe R, Stein DG. Morphologic features of embryonic neocortex grafts in adult rats following frontal cortical ablation. Brain Res 1987;401:162–67.
78. Stein DG, Labbe R, Attella MJ, Rakowsky H. Fetal brain tissue transplants reduce visual deficits in adult rats with bilateral lesions of the occipital cortex. Behav Neural Biol 1985;44:226–77.
79. Marciano FF, Wiegand SJ, Sladek JR Jr, Gash DM. Fetal hypothalamic transplants promote survival and functional regeneration of axotomized adult supraoptic magnocellular neurons. Brain Res, in press.

Chapter 2

The Importance of Clinical Data in the Treatment of Brain Injury

Brian T. Andrews
Lawrence H. Pitts

Despite the increasing use of sophisticated diagnostic and monitoring techniques, the clinical examination remains the simplest, most reliable, and most important tool for evaluating brain-injured patients [1]. The initial neurological examination provides information that may not only direct immediate management [2–4], but may also be of prognostic importance [3–14]. Subsequent neurological examinations may detect changes indicating a delayed complication of brain injury, such as intracerebral [15,16] or extracerebral [17] hematomas, and lead to further diagnostic studies and treatment. This chapter reviews the uses and limitations of the clinical examination during the initial evaluation and subsequent management of the brain-injured patient.

INITIAL EVALUATION

At San Francisco General Hospital, all patients with a suspected brain injury are evaluated upon arrival in the emergency room by a multispecialty trauma team, including a member of the Neurosurgical Service. While the extent of systemic injuries is being established and resuscitation is begun as needed, a neurological examination is performed and the results are recorded on a standardized form (Figure 2–1). The use of this form helps to prevent errors of omission and documents the neurological findings for comparison with subsequent examinations. Because severe systemic hypotension [18] or hypoxia [1,3] can lead to an abnormal neurological examination, these problems are corrected as promptly and completely as possible, and the examination is repeated. Blood pressure, pulse, and pulmonary function are monitored closely for deterioration that may affect neurological function. A urine sample is

SAN FRANCISCO GENERAL HOSPITAL

INPATIENT

PROGRESS RECORD

DATE TIME	PROBLEM NUMBER	FORMAT: PROBLEM NUMBER AND TITLE: S—Subjective O—Objective A—Analysis P—Plans			
		NEUROSURGICAL HEAD INJURY ADMITTING SHEET			
		Sex: ☐ Male / ☐ Female Age: Handedness: ☐ Left / ☐ Right			
		Cause of Injury:			
		Time from: Injury ➞ Coma Injury ➞ MEH Injury ➞ Neuro Consult			
	Physical Exam	Vital Signs BP HR TEMP			

COMA SCORE	GROUP A				GROUP B (Any circled area places patient in this group)		
Eye Opening	None				To pain	To voice	Spontaneously
Verbal Response	None	Garbled Sounds			Inappro. Words	Confused	Oriented
Motor Response	Flaccid	Abnormal Extension	Abnormal Flexion	Withdraws	Localizes Pain		Follows Command

MOTOR EXAM:

	R	L
arms		
legs		

1 = no response
2 = abnormal extension
3 = abnormal flexion
4 = weakness
5 = normal

Spontaneous spasms (posturing)? ☐ Yes / ☐ No

PUPILS: Ⓡ Size _____ mm Reaction + / −   Ⓛ Size _____ mm Reaction + / −

EOMs: III nerve palsy? ☐ Right   ☐ Left   ☐ Neither   ☐ Both

Spontaneous eye movements? Describe:

Doll's eyes: ☐ Absent   ☐ Sluggish   ☐ Brisk   ☐ Normal (awake)

Calorics: ☐ None   ☐ Dysconj.   ☐ Conj.   ☐ Nystagmus (BEST RESPONSE EITHER EAR)

CORNEALS: Right + / −   Left + / −

RESPIRATIONS: ☐ Regular   ☐ Ataxic   ☐ Periodic (Cheyne-Stokes)

Apneic? ☐ Yes ☐ No   Resp. Rate:

Cough? ☐ Yes ☐ No   Gag? ☐ Yes ☐ No

F 726N Rev. 9/77

Figure 2.1   Form used to record the neurological findings and Glasgow Coma Score at hospital admission for comparison with the results of subsequent examinations.

obtained to screen for alcohol, opiate, barbiturate, or other drug intoxication that could affect neurological function [1,19]. Elevated serum osmolality in an otherwise healthy trauma patient gives an estimate of ethanol intoxication. Serum electrolytes, blood urea nitrogen, creatinine, and liver function are also measured because each of them, if abnormal, may falsely depress neurological function [20]. Hypothermia, especially below 29°C, may also affect neurological function[9]; therefore, the neurological examination should be repeated as the patient is rewarmed. The detection and correction of these metabolic and physical factors may take time but must not delay the evaluation and treatment of correctable intracranial lesions. A lateral roentgenogram of the cervical spine is routinely obtained because cervical spinal cord injury may affect the sensory and motor functions of the extremities, rendering the neurological examination inaccurate in reflecting a deficit due to brain injury.

In a patient with altered consciousness, the examiner must assess responsiveness to verbal or painful stimuli and test brain stem reflexes [1]. Even though detailed tests of sensation, visual fields, and higher cortical function may not be possible, the examiner must accurately differentiate among neurological conditions ranging from mild neurological deficits to brain death. The Glasgow Coma Score (GCS) [21] is a reliable measure of the level of consciousness that is easy to use, is reproducible between observers [22], and has a powerful prognostic value as a measure of the severity of brain injury [11]. The GCS is recorded as part of the initial examination and monitored continuously during subsequent management.

At our institution, any patient with a severe brain injury, defined as a GCS of 8 or less (no eye opening, unable to speak or follow motor commands), is intubated, hyperventilated to produce an arterial carbon dioxide tension of 25–30 torr, and given intravenous mannitol (1–1.5 g/kg). Patients who are thrashing uncontrollably may be paralyzed and intubated to facilitate management. Subsequent steps in treating comatose brain-injured patients are dependent on the brain stem reflexes. If brain stem function is intact and the vital signs are stable, computerized tomographic (CT) brain scanning is performed immediately, and management is dictated by the results. CT scanning is also performed in patients with a history of brain trauma and possible drug overdose or in those with hypothermia or other metabolic abnormalities that may falsely depress results of the neurological examination [20].

Diagnostic Burr-Hole Placement

For many years, we have performed immediate bilateral burr-hole exploration before CT scanning in all patients with a clear history of brain injury who have clinical evidence of tentorial herniation or upper brain stem dysfunction. Patients in whom burr holes disclose an extracerebral hematoma undergo an immediate craniotomy to evacuate the clot; those without apparent hematoma undergo CT scanning immediately after burr-hole placement. In our recently published series [27], surgically significant extracerebral mass lesions were discovered by burr-hole exploration in 56 of 100 consecutive patients; in 38 patients, results of the exploration were negative, and postoperative CT scanning showed no significant hematomas [2]. In six patients with negative burr-hole explorations, postoperative CT scans demonstrated an extra-axial hematoma that required surgical evacuation. Four had subdural hematomas that were missed because the initial exploration, being limited to a single temporal burr hole, was incomplete. Two had hematomas (one subdural and one epidural) contralateral to a positive initial burr-hole exploration and subsequent craniotomy. Overall, 62 of these 100 patients had significant extra-axial hematomas amenable to immediate surgical diagnosis and evacuation. Intracerebral hematomas were missed during the initial surgical exploration in only three patients (3%); in two of them, however, an overlying subdural clot had been detected and immediately evacuated [2].

The mean age of patients with positive burr-hole exploration was 45.3 years. Falls (41%) and vehicle-pedestrian accidents (33%) were the most common causes of injury. Patients in whom burr-hole exploration was negative were younger (mean age, 35 years; $P < 0.001$) and most often were injured in motor vehicle accidents. Only 36% of patients younger than 30 years of age had positive burr-hole explorations, compared with 60% of those aged 30 to 59 years and 75% of those aged 60 years and older (chi square $= 8.26$, $P < 0.025$). Mass lesions were detected on the side of the initial exploration in 48 of 56 patients (86%). The initial burr hole was on the side of a single dilated pupil in 33 patients and on the side of obvious external brain trauma in 2 patients without lateralizing neurological signs.

These results support our belief that brain-injured patients with early clinical signs of tentorial herniation or upper brain stem compression need not undergo immediate CT scanning. The clinical examination in these patients most often indicates mechanical compression of the brain stem by an extra-axial hematoma, and immediate diagnostic and therapeutic burr-hole exploration is therefore indicated. Because significantly fewer extra-axial hematomas are found in patients younger than 30 years of age, especially those injured as motor vehicle occupants, these patients now undergo immediate CT scanning rather than exploratory burr-hole placement.

The decision to perform immediate exploratory burr holes depends on the initial neurological examination. Therefore, it is imperative that the clinical findings reflect intracranial pathology as accurately as possible. We perform diagnostic burr-hole exploration only if the patient has a clear history or obvious external evidence of brain injury. CT scans are obtained in comatose patients when the history of traumatic brain injury is in doubt or when clinical signs of brain stem dysfunction may be primarily due to central nervous system (CNS) depression from other causes, such as hypothermia, drug ingestion, or hypoxia [20].

Effects of Systemic Hypotension on the Neurological Examination

One group in which there is doubt concerning the validity of the neurological examination is brain-injured patients who have multiple injuries and systemic hypotension. At what degree of systemic hypotension does an abnormal neurological examination reflect brain ischemia from lack of perfusion rather than true brain injury or mechanical brain stem compression? To answer this question, we reviewed a series of 36 patients with documented brain injury, clinical signs of upper brain stem compression, and various degrees of systemic hypotension. All had had exploratory burr-hole placement for the diagnosis and treatment of intracranial hematomas [18]. On arrival in the emergency room, 10 patients were resuscitated from cardiac arrest, 7 had severe hypotension (systolic blood pressure [SBP] less than 60 torr), and 19 had moderate hypotension (SBP, 60–90 torr). The median initial GCS was 3 (range, 3–8). Although 4 of the 10 patients resuscitated from cardiac arrest had anisocoria, only 1 (10%) had an intracranial hematoma discovered at surgery. Only two of the seven patients with initially severe hypotension had anisocoria, and neither had an intracranial hematoma; one patient in this group (14%) had a small hematoma that was diagnosed at autopsy. In contrast, in 13 (68%) of the 19 patients with moderate hypotension and signs of tentorial herniation, intracranial hematomas were discovered at burr-hole placement; these 13 included 7 of the 9 patients (78%) found to have anisocoria on initial examination. In each of the latter patients, the hematoma was ipsilateral to the larger pupil. Thus, hematomas were more significantly frequent ($P < 0.05$), especially in the presence of anisocoria ($P < 0.01$), in patients with an initial SBP of 60 torr or greater than in those with an initially lower blood pressure.

These results suggest that in patients with moderate systemic hypotension, clinical evidence of anisocoria or upper brain stem dysfunction reflects mechanical compression of the brain stem by a mass lesion. We continue to evaluate such patients with immediate exploratory burr-hole placement rather than initial CT scanning. In patients with initial cardiac arrest or severe hypotension, however, brain stem dysfunction rarely indicates a mass lesion and more likely reflects brain stem ischemia. We prefer to evaluate such patients with CT scanning after initial resuscitation and stabilization. If an emergency laparotomy or thoracotomy is required for systemic injuries, exploratory burr holes are placed concurrently to diagnose and evacuate mass lesions regardless of the severity of systemic hypotension. We also begin to monitor the intracranial pressure (ICP) in the operating room while other surgery is being completed.

In all patients who undergo initial exploratory burr-hole placement, an ICP monitor (a subdural or intraventricular catheter) is placed intraoperatively. The ICP is continuously monitored during subsequent management as an adjunct to the clinical examination. Therefore, even among patients in whom the results of exploration are negative, we establish early ICP monitoring and treatment.

Throughout early therapy, the neurological examination should be repeated often, initially at hourly intervals. Even if a CT scan is negative soon after injury, there may be delayed development of an intra- or extra-axial hematoma [2,16,17]. Clinical deterioration should prompt immediate diagnostic reevaluation. In patients with a normal or near-normal neurological examination after initial unconsciousness (the classic "lucid interval"), progressive neurological deterioration can indicate an extra-axial hematoma [4,23] and warrants immediate repeat CT scanning. If the deterioration progresses to include signs of upper brain stem dysfunction, emergency burr-hole placement is indicated without CT scanning because of the high likelihood of an enlarging extra-axial hematoma.

SUBSEQUENT MANAGEMENT

The neurological examination is an essential tool for monitoring the clinical course of brain-injured patients after resuscitation, stabilization, diagnostic studies, and surgical intervention. Its most important function is to detect delayed intracerebral hematomas, which most often occur up to 24 hours after injury [16], recurrent hematomas [4], and cerebral edema [24]. A worsening of examination results may also reflect systemic complications, such as hypoxia or hypotension [3]. In our hospital, the neurological examination alone is monitored in patients with an initial GCS greater than 8. In these patients, changes in the level of consciousness are a sensitive indicator of such complications. In initially comatose patients (GCS of 8 or less), we rely on both the ICP and the neurological examination to guide clinical management. Complications such as hypoxia, systemic hypotension, and cerebral edema or hemorrhage in the temporal lobe may cause neurological deterioration without increasing ICP. In comatose patients, however, especially those with brain stem dysfunction, complications that lead to an increase in the ICP are not always accompanied by an evident neurological deterioration. We continuously monitor the blood pressure and pulse in the comatose brain-injured patient. Arterial hypotension, reflex bradycardia, or both (Cushing's reflex) may occasionally be the first sign of decreased perfusion of the brain stem. Because cerebral blood flow depends upon cerebral perfusion pressure (CPP), CPP is calculated by subtracting the ICP from the mean arterial pressure (CPP = MAP − ICP). Charting the vital signs, ICP, CPP, and neurological variables such as GCS and pupillary, corneal, and osculovestibular reflexes over time allows improvement or deterioration to be recognized.

Although the clinical examination and ICP monitoring are the primary means of detecting delayed complications of brain injury, the information they provide is by no means specific for guiding management. We rely heavily upon repeated CT scanning of the brain to evaluate patients who show clinical signs of deterioration. The rapid development of anisocoria or upper brain stem dysfunction is of particular concern because it may indicate a hematoma in the temporal lobe. Such a hematoma may occur without an increase in ICP and can result in severe morbidity if not rapidly diagnosed and evaluated. We recommend early CT scanning of any patient with new onset of anisocoria.

As during the initial clinical evaluation, the neurological examination may become unreliable if CNS-depressant medications (e.g., barbiturates) or paralytic agents are used or if significant hypothermia, hypoxia, or systemic hypotension develops [20]. Under these circumstances, the ICP should be monitored, and subsequent management should be guided by these values.

ICP monitoring is a useful indicator of neurological deterioration in the brain-injured patient [25,26], but the efficacy of monitoring and treating elevated ICP in reducing morbidity or mortality has not been demonstrated convincingly. Only the report of Bowers and Marshall has shown statistically improved survival among severely brain-injured patients (GCS of 5 or less) in whom the ICP was monitored and elevated ICP was treated, compared with similar patients in whom ICP was not monitored [7]. In a recent study of severely brain-injured patients, Smith et al found no difference in outcome between those treated with mannitol for ICP elevation greater than 25 torr and those who received empirical treatment with mannitol regardless of ICP readings [27]. Nevertheless, because increased ICP decreases cerebral perfusion, we attempt to keep it below 20 torr by administration of mannitol and hyperventilation. We try to maintain the cerebral perfusion pressure above 60 torr and use volume replacement with colloid or crystalloid fluids or, rarely, pressor agents to maintain normal mean arterial pressure.

DETERMINATION OF PROGNOSIS

The prognosis for patients with brain injuries is influenced by many factors, including the initial CT scan findings [28,29], the presence or absence of intracranial hematomas [4–7,23,30], uncontrolled elevation of ICP [6,7,26,31,32], and biochemical abnormalities [33]; but the most powerful predictors of outcome in these patients are the clinical data, including patient age, the presence of multiple injuries or systemic insults such as hypotension, and the early neurological examination. Numerous studies have demonstrated the relationship between the age of the patient and the outcome after brain injury [2,3,5,6,9,11–13]. In a review of 1,000 patients with severe brain injury who were divided into 5-year age groups, Jennett et al reported a steadily worsening prognosis for mortality or severe morbidity with increasing age [11]. Becker et al found mortality rates of 22% among patients less than 21 years of age and 57% among those over 60 years of age [5]. Gutterman and Shenkin showed that older patients were less able than younger patients to tolerate traumatic decerebration and have useful survival [10]. Recent reports of brain injury in children confirm that morbidity and mortality rates in these patients are lower than in adults [6,9]. Studies from our institution [2] and others [5,11] have shown that older brain-injured patients are more likely to harbor an intracranial hematoma, which worsens the prognosis in all age groups [4–9,11,23].

The presence of multiple injuries also worsens the prognosis after brain injury [3,13,34]. Overgaard et al reported that thoracic or abdominal injury and extremity fractures, alone or in combination, significantly reduced the survival rate among patients with moderate or severe brain injury; systemic hypertension (SBP $\geq$ 160 torr) correlated with increased morbidity and mortality rates in all age groups [13]. In a study by Miller et al, arterial hypotension, hypoxia, hypercarbia, and anemia were almost exclusively seen in patients with multiple systemic injuries in addition to severe brain injury and were associated with higher mortality and morbidity rates [3]. Systemic hypotension in patients with severe brain injury carries an extremely poor prognosis [3,18,34]. Newfield et al found that the mortality rate after severe brain injury increased from 45% in patients without initial hypotension to 83% (P < 0.001) in those with the same degree of brain injury and hypotension (SBO < 90 torr) during the first 24 hours of hospitalization [34]. In our series of 36 brain-injured patients with hypotension and signs of upper brain stem dysfunction, only 3 lived; each had mild hypotension that quickly responded to volume expansion. There were no survivors among those with initial cardiac arrest or severe hypotension (SBP < 60 torr) [18].

The most significant determinant of prognosis appears to be the severity of the primary brain injury as reflected by neurological examinations during the first several days [4,5,7,8,10,11,13,14]. The GCS has a major impact on morbidity and mortality rates. In their review of 1,000 patients, Jennett et al found that 82% of those whose best GCS was 11 or more within the first 24 hours had a moderate disability or a good recovery; 12% were vegetative or dead at the 6-month follow-up [11]. The outcome worsened steadily as the GCS decreased: among patients whose best GCS was 3 or 4 within the first 24 hours, only 7% had a moderate disability or a good recovery, and 87% were dead or vegetative at follow-up. Jennett et al emphasized that the initial neurological findings may be unduly pessimistic and that predictions based upon the best level of function during the first several days are most accurate [11]. Many other studies have confirmed the relationship of the early GCS to functional outcome [7,12,14] and have shown that it is a sensitive indicator even of subtle neuropsychological function, such as late cognitive outcome after brain injury [35].

Similarly, abnormalities of pupillary function, extraocular movement, and motor response indicate the severity of the primary brain injury and are predictors of poor recovery [4,5,8,10,11]. Bricolo et al reviewed 800 patients with severe brain injury and showed that, among patients with decerebrate (extensor) rigidity, only 16% achieved a functional recovery and 72% died. In contrast, patients with decorticate (flexor) rigidity or unilateral abnormal motor responses had better survival rates and functional outcome [8].

Prognostic data from the early neurological examination may be supplemented by the results of ICP monitoring [6,26,31,32]. In a study of 160 severely brain injured patients, Miller et al found that nearly half of those who died had severely elevated ICP at admission and that even mild elevation of ICP was associated with increased morbidity; however, among patients with normal ICP at admission the mortality rate was only 14%, and in 78% there was a good outcome or a moderate disability [26]. Pitts et al reported a significant linear relationship between the ICP at 6–24 hours after injury and the outcome at 3 months [31]. Bowers and Marshall reported statistically improved survival among patients with an initial GCS of 3–5 in whom ICP was monitored and treated, compared with similarly injured patients in whom ICP was not monitored [7]. Thus, it appears that ICP monitoring may supplement data obtained by neurological examination in determining the prognosis of severely injured patients and that treatment of elevated ICP may influence the outcome in some patient populations.

SUMMARY

Although sophisticated diagnostic tests, particularly CT scanning of the brain, are an important aspect of the initial evaluation and subsequent management of the brain-injured patient, the neurological examination is the most critical guide to immediate diagnostic and therapeutic intervention. Patients over 30 years of age in whom there is clinical evidence of upper brain stem compression after brain injury often have extra-axial hematomas; in these patients, we perform immediate exploratory burr-hole placement before CT scanning. The neurological findings accurately reflect intracranial pathology, such as expanding mass lesions, in hypotensive patients whose SBP is greater than 60 torr, but not in more severely hypotensive patients, most likely because of the effects of cerebral ischemia. The neurological examination remains the most important guide to treatment throughout the clinical course of the brain-injured patient. In comatose patients, concurrent ICP monitoring provides important additional information, especially if there are significant systemic injuries or if CNS-depressant medications or paralyzing agents are administered. Clinical data, including age, systemic injuries, and the neurological findings during the first 24 to 48 hours after brain injury remain the best predictors of final outcome. ICP monitoring may provide supplementary prognostic data, and treatment of ICP may improve outcome in selected patient groups.

REFERENCES

1. Pitts LH. Neurological evaluation of the head injury patient. Clin Neurosurg 1981;29:203–24.
2. Andrews BT, Pitts LH, Lovely, MP, Bartkowski H. Is computed tomographic scanning necessary in patients with tentorial herniation? Results of immediate

surgical exploration without computed tomography in 100 patients. Neurosurgery 1986;19:408–13.

3. Miller JD, Sweet RC, Narayan R, Becker DP. Early insults to the injured brain. JAMA 1978;240:439–42.

4. Stone JL, Rifai R, Sugar O, Lang RGR, Oldershaw JB, Moody RA. Subdural hematomas. 1. Acute subdural hematoma: progress in definition, clinical pathology and therapy. Surg Neurol 1983;19:216–31.

5. Becker DP, Miller JD, Ward JD, Greenberg RP, Young HF, Sakalas R. The outcome from severe head injury with early diagnosis and intensive management. J Neurosurg 1977;47:491–502.

6. Berger MS, Pitts LH, Lovely MP, Edwards MSB, Bartkowski HM. Outcome from severe head injury in children and adolescents. J Neurosurg 1985;62:194–99.

7. Bowers SA, Marshall LF. Outcome in 200 consecutive cases of severe head injury treated in San Diego County: A prospective analysis. Neurosurgery 1980;6:237–41.

8. Bricolo A, Turazzi S, Alexandre A, Rizzuto N. Decerebrate rigidity in acute head injury. J Neurosurg 1977;47:680–96.

9. Bruce DA, Schut L, Bruno LA, Wood JH, Sutton LN. Outcome following severe head injuries in children. J Neurosurg 1978;48:679–88.

10. Gutterman P, Shenkin HA. Prognostic features in recovery from traumatic decerebration. J Neurosurg 1970;32:330–35.

11. Jennett B, Teasdale G, Braakman R, Minderhound J, Heiden J, Kurze T. Prognosis of patients with severe head injury. Neurosurgery 1979;4:283–88.

12. Lokkeberg AR, Grimes RM. Assessing the influence of non-treatment variables in a study of outcome from severe head injury. J Neurosurg 1984;61:254–62.

13. Overgaard J, Hvid-Hansen O, Land AM, Pedersen KK, Christensen S, Haase J, Hein O, Tweed WA. Prognosis after head injury based on early clinical examination. Lancet 1973;2:631–35.

14. Williams JM, Gomes F, Drudge OW, Kessler M. Predicting outcome from closed head injury by early assessment of trauma severity. J Neurosurg 1984;61:581–85.

15. D'Avella D, De Blasi F, Rotilio A, Pensabene V, Pandolfo N. Intracerebral hematoma following evacuation of chronic subdural hematomas. J Neurosurg 1986;65:710–12.

16. Soloniuk D, Pitts LH, Lovely M, Bartkowski H. Traumatic intracerebral hematomas: Timing of appearance and indications for operative removal. J Trauma 1986;26:787–93.

17. Bucci MN, Phillips TW, McGillicudy JE. Delayed epidural hemorrhage in hypotensive multiple trauma patients. Neurosurgery 1986;19:65–68.

18. Andrews BT, Levy ML, Pitts LH. The implications of systemic hypotension for the neurological examination in patients with severe head injury. Surg Neurol 1987;28:419–22.

19. Jagger J, Fife D, Vernberg K, Jane JA. Effect of alcohol intoxication on the diagnosis and apparent severity of brain injury. Neurosurgery 1984;15:303–6.

20. Pitts LH. Determination of brain death. West J Med 1984;140:628–31.

21. Teasdale G, Jennett B. Assessment of coma and impaired consciousness: A practical scale. Lancet 1974;2:81–84.

22. Teasdale G, Knill-Jones R, Van der Sorder J. Observer variability in assessing impaired consciousness and coma. J Neurol Neurosurg Psychiatr 1978;41:603–10.

23. Marshall LF, Toole BM, Bowers SA. The national traumatic coma data bank. 2.

Patients who talk and deteriorate: Implications for treatment. J Neurosurg 1983; 59:285–88.

24. Ropper AH. Lateral displacement of the brain and level of consciousness in patients with an acute hemispheral mass. N Engl J Med 1986;314:953–58.

25. Galbraith S, Teasdale G. Predicting the need for operation in the patient with an occult traumatic intracranial hematoma. J Neurosurg 1981;55:75–81.

26. Miller JD, Becker DP, Ward JD, Sullivan HG, Adams WE, Rosner MJ. Significance of intracranial hypertension in severe head injury. J Neurosurg 1977;47:503–16.

27. Smith HP, Kelly DL, McWhorter JM, Armstrong D, Johnson R, Transou C, Howard G. Comparison of mannitol regimens in patients with severe head injury undergoing intracranial monitoring. J Neurosurg 1986;65:820–24.

28. Lobato RD, Sarabia R, Rivas JJ, Cordobes F, Castro S, Munoz MJ, Cabrera A, Barcena A, Lamas E. Normal computerized tomography scans in severe head injury. J Neurosurg 1986;65:784–89.

29. Toutant SM, Klauber MR, Marshall LF, Toole BM, Bowers SA, Seelig JM, Varnell JB. Absent or compressed basal cisterns on fast CT scan: Ominous predictors of outcome in severe head injury. J Neurosurg 1984;61:691–94.

30. Gennarelli TA, Spielman GM, Langfitt TW, Gildenberg PL, Harrington T, Jane JA, Marshall LF, Miller JD, Pitts LH. Influence of the type of intracranial lesion on outcome from severe head injury. A multicenter study using a new classification system. J Neurosurg 1982;56:26–32.

31. Pitts LH, Katkis JV, Juster R, Heilbron D. ICP and outcome in patients with severe head injury. In: Shulman K, Marmarou A, Miller J, Becker D, Hockwald GM, Brock M, eds. Intracranial pressure. New York: Springer-Verlag, 1980;5–8.

32. Uzzell BP, Obrist WD, Dolinska CA, Langfitt TW. Relationship of acute CBF and ICP findings to neuropsychological outcome in severe head injury. J Neurosurg 1986;65:630–35.

33. DeSalles AAF, Kontos HA, Becker DP, Yang MS, Ward JD, Moutlon R, Gruemer HD, Lutz H, Maset A, Jenkins L, Marmarou A, Muizelaar P. Prognostic significance of ventricular CSF lactic acidosis in severe head injury. J Neurosurg 1986;65:615–24.

34. Newfield P, Katkis L, Hoff J, Boggan J. Influence of shock on survival after head injury. Neurosurgery 1980;6:596–97.

35. Alexandre A, Colombo F, Nertempi P, Benedetti A. Cognitive outcome and early indices of severity of head injury. J Neurosurg 1983;59:751–61.

Chapter 3

Technology in the Management of Head Injury

Bryan Jennett

The British approach to medical management of head injuries generally stresses bare-hands clinical observation, whereas the American approach relies more on technology. My position as an advocate for, or at least reviewer of, technology compels me to stop and think what song to sing, rather than rehearsing a well-worn tune from a standard repertoire. We must consider the overall perspective of technology in the management of head injuries in the acute stage. Certain questions need to be asked before we add a new technology to the "have-to-have" list and it becomes a "has-to-be-paid-for" item.

For me, *technology* means tools that enhance our ability to perform the tasks of medicine—diagnosis, monitoring, prognosis, and treatment. The two main types of technology are those that provide information and those that are interventions. Some information must be collected before decisions can be made about the need to seek more information from investigations in order to decide about the need for therapeutic interventions. Information may also be useful in adding to our store of knowledge and our breadth of understanding. It should, however, be clearly recognized and acknowledged when the purpose of seeking data is an academic one.

Interventions may be directed toward minimizing adverse factors that can threaten life or impede recovery, or toward actively maximizing recovery. Because we know little about how brain function is restored after injury, most interventions are of the former two kinds. We aim to reduce the risks that complications will cause additional damage to the brain, by attempting to predict, anticipate, prevent, recognize, or treat these complications.

Trauma to the head differs from that to other parts of the body in that most effort is devoted to dealing with secondary events, whereas little can be done about the damage to the brain sustained at the time of the injury. Elsewhere in the body, damage is normally maximal at onset and active repair is required of the surgeon, whether fixing a fracture, stabilizing the chest wall, restoring continuity to torn gut or lacerated liver, or replacing degloved skin. Apart from debridement and closure of a compound depressed fracture of the skull, neurosurgeons dealing with recent head injury have no immediate restorative interventions in their operative repertoire. This makes head trauma technically unattractive to neurosurgeons.

The adverse secondary developments that we seek to counter are of two kinds, intracranial and extracranial. Inside the head there may be a hematoma or brain swelling, with consequent raised intracranial pressure (ICP) and reduced blood flow. A much less common risk is infection. Extracranial complications with implications for the brain include blood loss, hypotension, hypoxia, raised intrathoracic pressure and, if coma persists, inadequate nutrition.

Rational decisions depend on reliable data about what *has* happened (diagnosis), what *is* happening now (monitoring), and what *will* happen in the near and distant future (prognosis). Technologies for head injury can therefore be listed under several categories. Both the skull and the brain may be visualized or imaged in various ways. Physiological functions can be measured, including cardiorespiratory, ICP, and brain activity. The various data yielded by technological diagnostic and monitoring techniques can then be processed along with data from clinical observations and the patient's age. This requires another technology, that of the microchip, leading to the possibility of computer-assisted diagnosis and prognosis as an aid to decision making.

Given that most of the technologies are in the diagnostic/monitoring modes, it is appropriate to consider the general principles that should inform their provision and use [1]. The basic questions are: do we need to know, or would it be nice to know? In other words, is it action-oriented or academic? Need to know carries, of course, a sliding scale of benefits and burdens. Obvious benefits are that positive findings may indicate the likely course of events, and so contribute to appropriate management decisions. But negative findings can be equally useful, making it possible to avoid inappropriate interventions, such as unnecessary additional tests or monitoring, and unjustified therapies.

The burdens of newly available investigative technologies are that too many tests may be done; a degree of hazard and discomfort from invasive procedures; and the risk that false-positive results may precipitate unjustified further interventions, either tests or therapy. Such false positives may derive from limitations of equipment or of interpretation.

The impact of an innovative diagnostic technology may therefore be to improve the process of diagnosis by reducing the discomfort, risk, or expense of investigative procedures. Quite separately, it may improve the accuracy of diagnosis, providing information of a kind not previously available. This information may influence management decisions, but the real test of the effectiveness of a technology is whether it favorably influences patient outcome. Some radiologists have rejected this as an unrealistic goal. Meanwhile, commentators have raised the suspicion that some diagnostic and monitoring technologies do more to improve the quality of life of the doctors who use them than of the patients subjected to them, at least until the doctors learn to deploy them appropriately.

A good example of this was the delay before it was shown that CT scanning had a favorable influence on the *outcome* of head injured patients who reached regional neurosurgical units in the United Kingdom. When results were reviewed some four years after this technology had been introduced, everyone trumpeted its benefits; they had been able to abandon emergency angiography and the use of exploratory burr holes, or "woodpecker surgery." The pejorative overtones of this term may have to be revised in the light of the work of Andrews and Pitts (see Chapter 2). According to them, some patients who arrive at a neurosurgical service with clear clinical evidence of advanced cerebral compression can be salvaged by immediate surgery. For these few patients, the delay associated with securing a CT scan may reduce the chance of survival or of reasonable recovery. Andrews and Pitts emphasize that their recommendation applies only when an operating room can be mobilized more rapidly than a CT scan can be completed.

In the late 1970s, three large neurosurgical units (in London, Glasgow, and Liverpool) each reported their disappointment that hospital mortality seemed unchanged since the introduction of CT scanning [2–4]. In Glasgow we realized that the most likely reason was that the criteria for transfer to a regional unit for specialist investigation had not been changed. Doctors appeared still to be waiting for a high index of suspicion that an intracranial hematoma had already developed; this had been customary before submitting patients to the hazards of angiography.

When in Glasgow we deliberately changed the policy for transfer, the number of patients sent each year to the neurosurgical unit for CT scanning doubled. This new policy also ensured that scanning was done sooner after injury, and that the condition of fewer patients deteriorated seriously before surgery. More importantly, the number of surgically significant hematomas discovered each year almost doubled, and postoperative mortality and morbidity improved. It is important to realize that this new policy required a change of attitude and behavior on the part of doctors in disciplines other than neurosurgery and neuroradiology, of doctors who mostly work in hospitals other than those where these specialities were practiced. This indicates that even the most efficacious technology cannot be effective for the community at large if it is not used appropriately.

As CT scanners begin to be available in more and more district (or community) hospitals in Britain, some are warning of the threat of a different kind of inappropriate use. It seems likely that some patients in need of urgent neurosurgical care may suffer delay while an inexpert scan is done before transfer. In some places the scan may have to be repeated at the neurosurgical unit to provide data of adequate quality for the surgeon. In other patients there will be false-positive results. At best these patients will have an unnecessary transfer; at worst they may find themselves under the knife of an enthusiastic trauma surgeon who has difficulty in controlling intracranial bleeding and inflicts additional brain damage. This is a problem not only for Britain, because neurosurgical services are similarly regionalized throughout Europe, in Australia, and in many other countries.

The criteria for the appropriate *use* of a diagnostic technology depend on the answers to a number of questions [1]. Is there a reasonable probability of detecting a significant abnormality? What is the cost of detection, not just financially but in terms of risk, discomfort, and inconvenience? What are the benefits of detecting or of excluding the specific abnormality being sought? What are the consequences of failure to detect? The questions about *provision* are: What data are provided by this technology and of what value are these to patients? Which patients, and therefore how many patients, stand to benefit? Based on this estimate, how many machines should there be?

These questions take on a slightly different flavor when applied to *monitoring*. Remember the Oxford English Dictionary definition of a monitor: "a lizard that gives warning of approaching crocodiles." This implies that it is action-oriented. Critics of general, postoperative, and coronary intensive care units (ICUs) in the United States have emphasized that only a small proportion of patients who are admitted ever develop problems or require interventions. The questions, therefore, are: What is the probability that a complication will develop? What are the benefits of detecting this in the ICU rather than on the ward floor? What are the risks of monitoring, per se, when it involves invasive procedures? What are the risks of inappropriate interventions activated by the results of monitoring?

Many fewer tools are available for the *treatment* of head injuries. There is surgery, substituting natural ventilation and nutrition, intensive nursing care, and the use of drugs to control raised ICP or to reduce oxygen demand by the damaged brain. However, therapeutic technologies lend themselves to much more direct evaluation. The questions are: Does the procedure in question produce a significantly better outcome than was predicted, and does it do so in a significant number of patients? That begs the question of how to define outcome and to value it, as well as how reliably it can be predicted.

Based on patient age, and on the severity of both the injury and the physiological abnormality, it is now possible to predict outcome in broad terms in many patients. This was shown by the Glasgow/Netherlands study 10 years ago [5] and subsequently confirmed in the Glasgow/California studies [6–10]. This has subsequently been confirmed by Knaus of Washington for general ICUs in different states [11] and between hospitals in the United States and France [12]. All of these studies have revealed wide variations in the details of management in different places. Yet the outcome for groups of patients matched for features that influence outcome is similar. Indeed, the outcome of groups of patients in one center can be accurately predicted on the basis of cases collected elsewhere where management is different.

This does not, as some critics have asserted, imply a doctrine of therapeutic nihilism. All the patients in these studies were treated with vigor in first-class units that had the resolve and strength of character to take on the discipline of data collection required for participation in multicenter studies. That more than one-third of severely brain-injured patients recovered their independence (good or moderate on the Glasgow outcome scale) is a tribute to timely surgery for intracranial hematomas in some cases and to skillful intensive care for all of these patients, each of whom was in coma for at least six hours. It also indicates that various additional interventions, used much more often in some centers than others, do not seem to have significantly influenced outcome when patients with a similar prognosis are compared. There are, however, selected patients for whom one or more such techniques may be of benefit. The art of evaluating a therapy is to discover the sliding scale of benefits and burdens that define the limits of appropriate use, thus discovering which patients are likely to benefit.

Once the sliding scale has been defined and agreed upon, written guidelines or a protocol may be useful. Thus, when rapid decisions have to be made, often at unsocial hours and by junior staff, the actions taken will be consistent with a prior consensus. This will be in accord with the policy of senior clinicians who have weighed the evidence on the value of alternative actions and have reached conclusions about their appropriate use. Such a policy must be kept under constant review in the light of experience. This means formal, on-going audit rather than reliance on clinical impressions.

The use of predictions, both for management and for evaluation, can be considered in this way. If calculations indicate that a reasonable recovery is highly probable by reason of patient age and severity of injury, then certain elaborate interventions may not be justified because they are unnecessary. Per contra, if death or vegetative survival is predicted with confidence, then interventions would be unjustified because they are bound to be unsuccessful. This leaves the patients for whom the outcome is uncertain. It is on these patients that most therapeutic effort should be expended, and they should also be the focus of evaluations of new or existing therapies. This is because a statistically satisfactory result is likely to be achieved with many fewer patients. The trial will not be contaminated by the many patients whose outcome, because of patient age and severity of injury, cannot be influenced.

There is evidence that neurosurgeons may be prepared to use such predictions when making decisions about brain-injured patients [13]. Reliable predictors of outcome would also make it more possible to put into practice the recommendation of ethicists that neurosurgeons be discriminating in the continued treatment of severely brain-injured patients who are unlikely to recover [14].

Concern is sometimes expressed that this utilitarian approach to the investigation, monitoring, and treatment of head injuries might impede the development of new methods that could prove valuable. That is to misread my message. On the diagnostic/monitoring side, let me remind you of my distinction between need to know (for action) and nice to know (for science or curiosity). My contention is that the use of expensive or invasive new technologies is justified only in the context of a carefully constructed protocol that will ensure that lessons about usefulness are learned rapidly and reliably. Such lessons are unlikely to be learned when individual radiologists, anesthetists, or surgeons embark on haphazard fishing expeditions with occasional patients, and translate their "experience" into anecdotal accounts of success.

Exactly the same goes for newly emerging therapies, whether based on newly minted technologies or drugs, or on novel combinations or applications of technologies and drugs already available. These innovations are justified only within the context of careful data collection and analysis. That does not necessarily mean the expense and ethical implications of a randomized trial. For it is increasingly acknowledged that, when evaluating complex regimes used for rapidly developing life-threatening conditions, such a trial may not always be the most appropriate tool. However, we should not revert to casual comparisons with historical controls. Instead we should collect data, systematically and prospectively, about severity and type of injury, about therapeutic modalities used, and about outcome. Only by these means can guidelines evolve for the appropriate use of technologies. What is appropriate in one place may not be in another, whether it be a different country or a different hospital.

REFERENCES

1. Jennett B. High technology medicine. Benefits and burdens. 2nd ed. New York: Oxford University Press, 1986.
2. Ambrose J, Gooding MR, Uttley D. EMI scan in the management of head injuries. Lancet 1973;1:847–49.
3. Jeffreys RV, Lozado L. The use of the CAT scanner in the management of patients with head injury transferred to the regional neurosurgical unit. Injury 1981;13:370–74.
4. Teasdale G, Galbraith S, Murray L, Ward P, Gentleman D, McKean M. Management of traumatic intracranial hematoma. Br Med J 1982;285:1695–97.
5. Jennett B, Teasdale G, Braakman R, Minderhoud J, Knill-Jones R. Predicting outcome in individual patients after severe head injury. Lancet 1976;1:1031–34.
6. Jennett B, Teasdale G, Braakman R, Minderhoud J, Heiden J, Kurze T. Prognosis of patients with severe head injury. Neurosurgery 1979;4:283–88.
7. Jennett B, Teasdale G, Fry J, Braakman R, Minderhoud J, Heiden J, Kurze T. Treatment for severe head injury. J Neurol Neurosurg Psychiatr 1980;43:289–95.
8. Jennett B. Outcome of intensive therapy for severe head injuries: an inter-center comparison. In: Parillo JE, Ayres SM, eds. Major issues in critical care medicine. Baltimore: Williams & Wilkins, 1984.
9. Murray GD. Use of an international data bank to compare outcome following severe head injury in different centres. Stat med 1986;5:103–12.
10. Murray GD, Murray LS, Barlow P, Teasdale GM, Jennett B. Assessing the performance and clinical impact of a computerised prognostic system in severe head injury. Stat Med 1986;5:403–10.
11. Knaus WA, LeGall JR, Wagner DP, Draper EA, Loirat P, Campos RA, Cullen DJ, Kohles MK, Glaser P, Granthil C, Mercier P, Nicolas F, Nikki P, Shin B, Snyder JV, Wattel F, Zimmerman JE. A comparison of intensive care in the USA and France. Lancet 1982;2:642–46.

12. Knaus WA, Draper EA, Wagner DP, Zimmerman JE, Birnbaum ML, Cullen DJ, Kohles MK, Shin B, Snyder JV. Evaluation outcome from intensive care: A preliminary multihospital comparison. Crit Care Med 1982;10:491–96.
13. Barlow P, Teasdale G. Prediction of outcome and the management of severe head injuries: The attitudes of neurosurgeons. Neurosurgery 1986;19:989–91.
14. Engelhardt HT Jr. Ensuring against tragedy: The decision to treat the severely head injured. In: Miner ME, Wagner KA, eds. Neurotrauma: treatment, rehabilitation and related issues. Boston: Butterworths, 1986.

Part II

Technology and Assessment of Brain Injury

Michael E. Miner

We work in a highly technological age. Technical advances often benefit patient care but sometimes befuddle the clinician and always seem expensive. Radiologists now offer some of the most expensive technology, but also, in selected cases, the most cost effective. CT scanning has not only revolutionized neurodiagnosis but has also proven to be one of the most cost-effective technologies for the brain-injured patient. But what of magnetic resonance imaging (MR)? Joel Yeakley et al provide evidence that MR can extend the diagnosis of lesions of the central nervous system far beyond CT. They also discuss some of the limitations of this technology. Certainly MR can detect more lesions earlier, but is this of value? Yes, even if it does no more than document abnormalities and trigger caution in making a prognosis. MR may also help in evaluating the distribution of medications into the brain. This exciting possibility, just now being explored, may provide extremely valuable information that can extend our decision making far beyond current limits.

Intracranial pressure (ICP) monitoring has been another highly visible technology used to monitor patients after injury. At this juncture, ICP monitoring has gained general acceptance, but it measures only one phenomenon that reflects on the really critical issue. For it is not ICP that we want to control, but rather the survival of neurons. Steven Allen describes how measurement of the brain's oxygen use can augment ICP monitoring, making it a better monitor of brain survival. In his scheme, oxygen use reflects whole-brain viability. One of the real values of this type of technology is that it can be applied with equipment currently available to most modern intensive care units and does not require dedicated laboratory personnel.

The entire basis of acute treatment is to increase the survival of neurons, maintain life, and limit nonneurologic disability. The role of treatment with hyperbaric oxygen has not been established because few institutions have access to it, and even when available it is a cumbersome technology. However, Gaylan Rockswold et al present fascinating data that suggest that hyperbaric oxygen treatment can yield a better quality of survival in some brain-injured patients. Their work should be explored because, although their findings are very encouraging, this remains a difficult management regimen. Even so, one cannot but be impressed with their dedication and with the results they have attained.

Seizures are a perplexing problem in brain-injured patients. They are frequent immediately after injury but are usually not a major problem in the acute care situation. However, the long-term sequela of epilepsy for these patients is immense. James Wilmore discusses the literature on the subject and concludes that treating seizure disorders is valuable but trying to prevent seizures by the currently available medications is questionable. The future is uncertain, but the problem of seizures in brain-injured patients will remain as will the need to test new treatment regimens.

Barbara Wilson et al discuss the problems of using neurocognitive evaluation in the real world. Does performance on a pegboard in a quiet room predict how well an individual will cope with grocery shopping? These investigators report on their experience in testing and training brain-injured individuals in "real-world" terms. Their report is truly a bright spot for the pragmatist in us all. They delve into an area to which all effort in brain injury treatment should be directed—living in the world.

Chapter 4

The Role of Magnetic Resonance Imaging in Head Trauma

Joel W. Yeakley
Golden Pan
Madan V. Kulkarni

When any new imaging modality is introduced, the usual procedure is to compare it with existing modalities. When comparing magnetic resonance imaging (MR) with CT, one must realize that MR images are not interpreted in terms of x-ray attenuation or in terms of radiographic density as are CT images. Instead of using Hounsfield units as in CT, one must learn to interpret the parameters of T_1 and T_2 relaxation times, flow phenomena, proton density, and chemical shift. These measure various physical and chemical properties of protons in a magnetic field modified by radiofrequency waves. The result is a digital image, the elements of which are recorded as signal intensity[1].

Normally, when MR images are printed on film and transilluminated, a low signal intensity will be perceived as dark or black, whereas a high signal intensity will be recorded as bright or white. A detailed discussion of T_1 and T_2 relaxation times may be found in any standard MR textbook. However, it is sufficient to say here that long T_1 and short T_2 relaxation times will be shown as black or low signal intensity, whereas short T_1 and long T_2 relaxation times will appear as white or high signal intensity.

Those who persist in thinking in terms of x-ray density or attenuation will remain confused about the interpretation of MR images. An American learning a foreign language initially translates every word into English. Eventually, however, this individual learns to connect the visualized object directly to the word in a foreign language. Similarly, anyone learning the metric system who continually tries to convert kilometers to miles will remain confused. The confusion disappears when one learns to think in terms of how far a kilometer is. Therefore, to interpret MR scans, one must learn to think in terms of MR parameters and how they relate to the physical and chemical properties of normal and pathologically altered brain, rather than constantly trying to relate the MR appearance to that of the CT.

The following are guidelines for interpreting conventional MR images [1,2].

Bright on a T_1 weighted image:

Fat/marrow

Blood (hematoma greater than 4 or 5 days old)

Protein-rich fluid (necrosis, abscess, "bound water")

Mucus

Melanin

Slow flow

Bright on T_2 weighted image:

Tumor

Gliosis

Edema

Blood (hematoma beyond the first week)

Fluid

Intervertebral disk

Dark on T_1 and T_2 weighted images

Air

Fast flow

Calcium

Iron (hemosiderin)

Blood (acute hematoma less than 7 days duration)

Ligaments and tendons

With this background in mind let us turn to general consideration of the use of MR and CT in the evaluation of acute brain trauma. At present, a CT scan of the brain can usually be accomplished in 5 or 10 minutes. A general evaluation of the brain by MR takes approximately 30 minutes with conventional scanning methods. The MR scanning time may decrease, however, with newer "fast-scan" techniques [3]. Although current life support and monitoring devices present no obstacle to CT scanning, they may be incompatible with MR. This is because ferromagnetic components can be pulled into the high-strength magnetic field or cause noise interference with radiofrequency pulse sequences. However, MR-compatible life support and monitoring devices are rapidly becoming available [2–4].

Several other factors may currently limit the use of MR for brain trauma. Because of shielding requirements, machine weight, cryogen accessibility needs, and other site-planning problems, MR magnets may not be in close proximity to the emergency department and emergency resuscitative facilities. Also, an MR evaluation of the brain costs about twice as much as a comparable CT scan. Furthermore, many hospitals to which a brain injury patient initially presents may not have access to MR, whereas CT units are now almost universally available. Finally, ferromagnetic material located in the head of a trauma patient may produce image degradation. There have been reports of neurologic injury secondary to movement of metallic fragments in the magnetic field [5].

Identifying acute extracerebral blood collections may be the most important reason for imaging in patients with acute trauma, because these can be surgically drained if necessary. Acute extracerebral blood collections (subdural and epidural hematomas) of surgically significant size can usually be identified by CT or MR. An acute subdural hematoma less than 3 mm thick might be missed with MR if it is isointense relative to brain parenchyma [6], or to the inner table of the skull. This would be unlikely, however, with multiple pulse sequences [6,7]. Small extracerebral hematomas, particularly in the subacute stage, are better seen with MR and may be missed on CT, especially in unusual locations such as in the subfrontal, subtemporal, peritentorial, or clival areas (Figures 4.1–4.3). Extracerebral hematomas in these locations sometimes mimic intraparenchymal lesions on CT, so that coronal scanning or reconstruction is necessary to differentiate the two. MR has the advantage of providing the sagittal and coronal planes without patient manipulation; these may also clarify the extent of extracerebral hematoma. MR is relatively free of artifact in the posterior fossa compared with CT, so the distribution of extracerebral hematomas in that area may be better defined [8]. The extracerebral hematomas were small in those instances where MR detected lesions that CT did not. It is possible that the additional information gained by MR would not affect the surgical treatment of the patient [6,8].

MR also offers further differentiation of epidural and subdural hematomas, in that a black line corresponding anatomically to the dura may be identified in epidural hematoma [8,9]. "Isodense" subdural hematomas may be difficult to detect with CT unless contrast is administered. These collections are easily detected by MR [7,9,10]. MR is capable of distinguishing subdural hygroma from chronic subdural hematoma and mixed subdural hematomas consisting of acute and chronic hemorrhage based on their differing T_1 and T_2 relaxation times [8,11].

Although skull fractures are sometimes detected by MR (Figure 4.4), it does not demonstrate bony injuries as well as CT does. This disadvantage may be important in depressed fractures, basal skull fractures, and associated facial

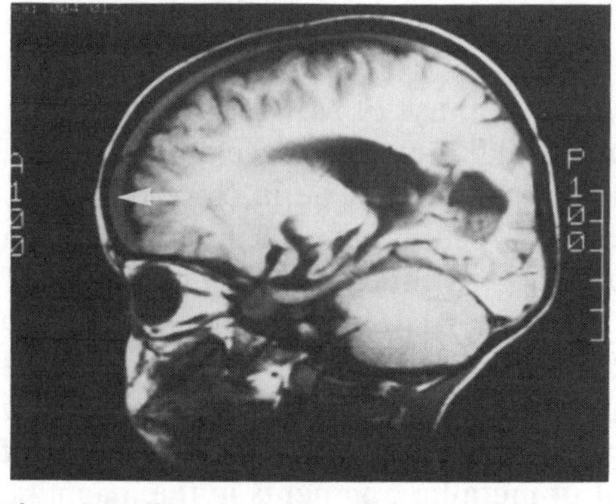

A

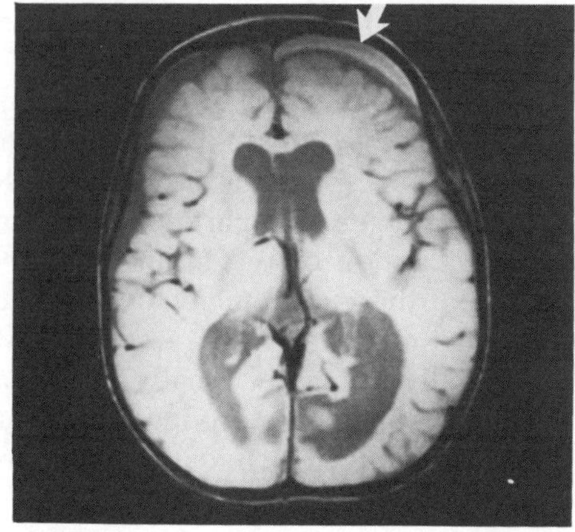

B

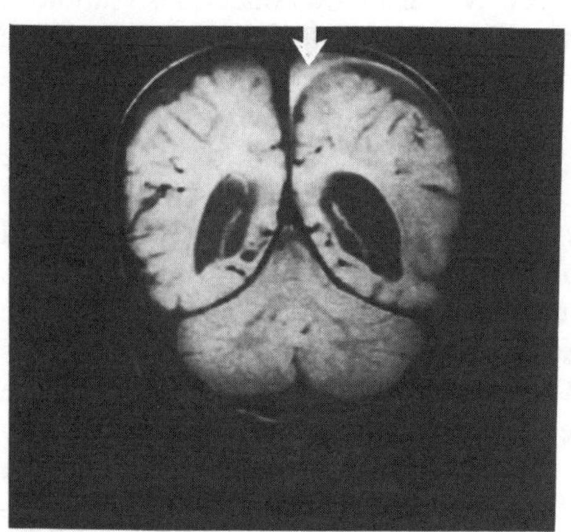

C

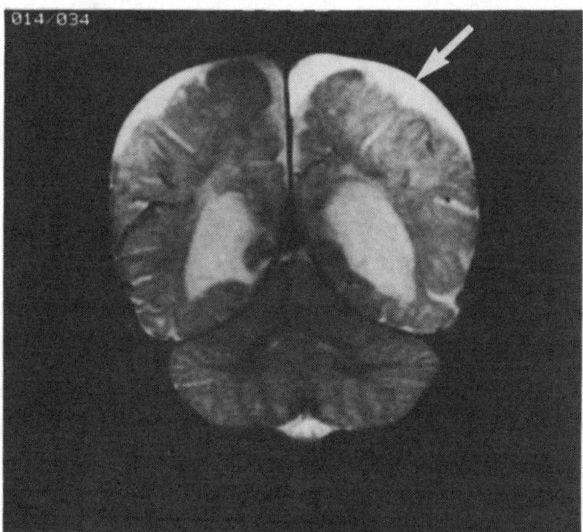

D

Figure 4.1   Subdural hematoma. (A) Sagittal T_1 weighted image shows subacute subdural hematoma as a gray zone (arrow) between the black-appearing skull and black appearing cerebrospinal fluid in the subarachnoid space. (B) Axial "proton density" MR confirms crescent-shaped subdural hematoma (arrow) in left frontal area. (C) Coronal "proton density" MR shows the white-appearing, crescent-shaped subacute subdural hematoma (arrow), which can be distinguished from the gray-appearing cerebrospinal fluid in the subarachnoid space. (D) T_2 weighted MR from same location as (B) demonstrates the subdural hematoma on the left (arrow), which is now more difficult to separate from the cerebrospinal fluid because both now appear white.

injuries [12,13]. However, MR may better visualize the soft tissue components of such injuries, for example, orbital blowout fractures [13].

Cortical contusions most frequently involve the inferior, lateral, and anterior aspects of the frontal and temporal lobes. Shearing injuries, however,

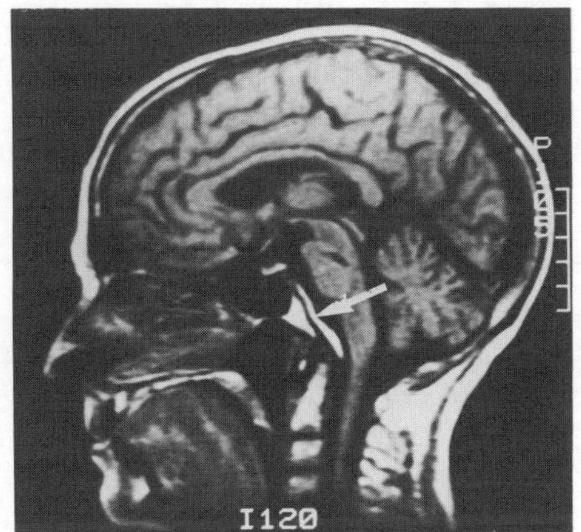

Figure 4.2 Clival subdural hematoma. Sagittal T_1 weighted MR shows subdural hematoma (arrow) along the clivus at the base of skull. This would be difficult if not impossible to recognize with CT.

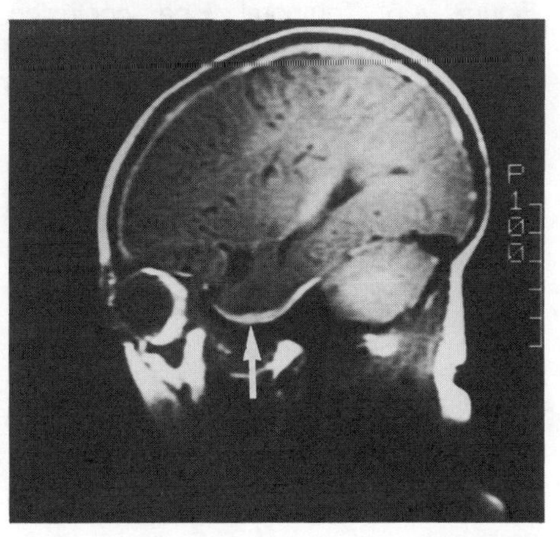

A

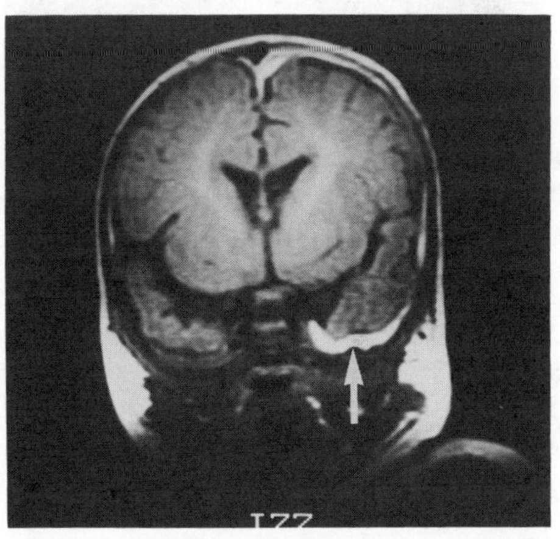

B

Figure 4.3 Subtemporal and convexity subdural hematomas. (A) Sagittal T_1 weighted MR shows subacute subdural hematoma below the temporal lobe (arrow). This is another location where blood collections are difficult to detect with CT. (B) Coronal T_1 weighted MR confirms subtemporal subdural hematoma (arrow) and shows another subdural hematoma over the vertex cerebral hemisphere on the same side.

are usually located more deeply at gray-white interfaces—particularly, adjacent to the internal capsule and fornix, corpus callosum, coronal radiata, and subcortical arcuate fibers (Figures 4.5 and 4.6). In regard to detection of these hemorrhagic contusions and shearing injuries, MR is quite sensitive in the acute phase when a complete sequence of conventional T_1 and T_2 weighted images is performed [14–17]. Acute clot produces low intensity on T_2 weighted images. Acute hemorrhage may be frequently isointense to brain on T_1 weighted

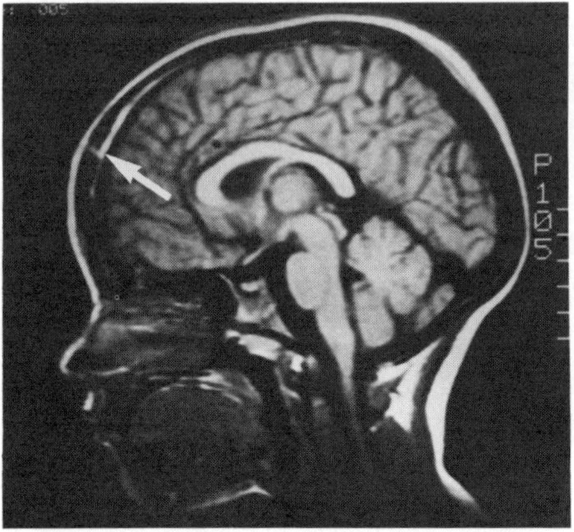

Figure 4.4 Frontal skull fracture with small subdural hematoma. Sagittal T_1 weighted MR shows fluid in fracture line (white) through the frontal bone (black). A small subacute hematoma (arrow) is seen beneath the fracture.

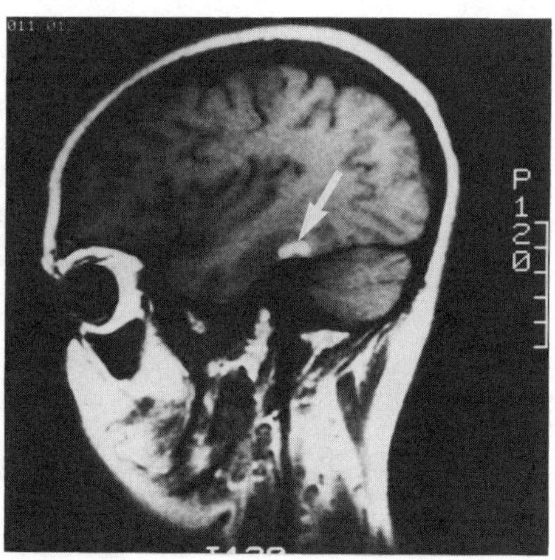

Figure 4.5 Temporal lobe contusion. Sagittal T_1 weighted MR shows an area of white-appearing increased signal intensity (arrow) in the left temporal lobe immediately above the black-appearing, triangle-shaped petrous ridge. Contusions in this location are difficult to detect by CT, due to artifact created by the adjacent bone.

sequences. Most acute hemorrhagic contusions are seen well on CT because of their increased density relative to brain tissue. Acute hemorrhage appears to be better detected by MR scanners with high field strength (1.5 tesla) than by those with lower field strength [2,6]. Newer "fast-scan" (gradient-recalled) techniques offer improvement in this regard because they are sensitive to the presence of blood products that cause detectable changes in magnetic susceptibility [3]. Whereas clotted blood undergoes rapid evolutionary change on CT that may make evaluation of hematomas and contusion difficult after a few weeks, the various degradation products of hemoglobin produce a more prolonged evolutionary process on MR, allowing follow-up of hematomas or hemorrhagic contusions for months or years (Figures 4.7–4.10).

Recent experience indicates that there are small amounts of hemorrhage detectable by MR that cannot be perceived on CT. As with hemorrhagic infarcts, these blood products are usually more easily detected by MR, espe-

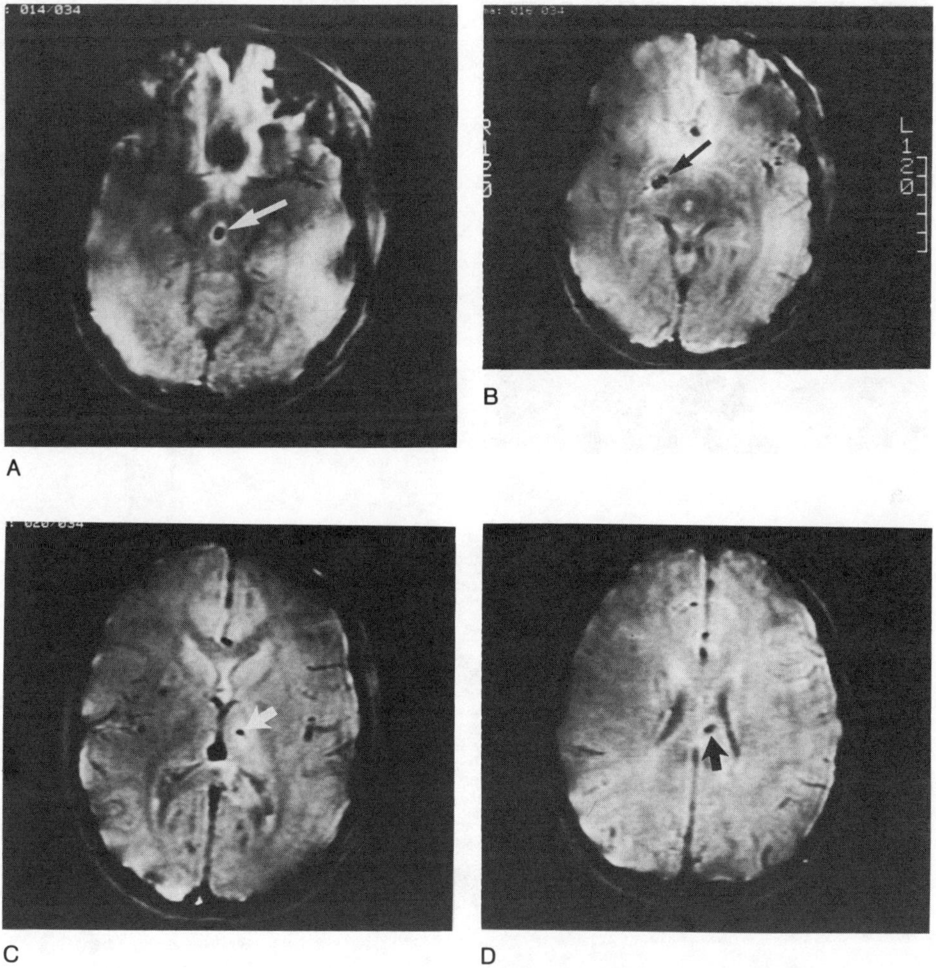

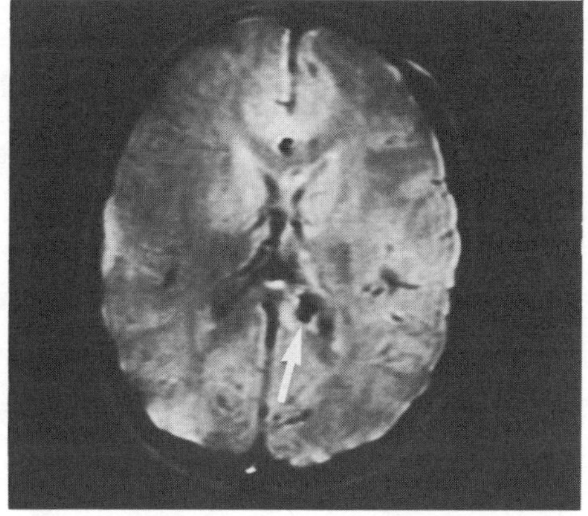

Figure 4.6 Multiple shearing injuries and brain stem hemorrhage. Axial "fast-scan" images, using gradient-recalled echo refocusing, show brain stem hemorrhage (A) and shearing injuries in the internal capsule (B), thalamus (C), and corpus callosum (D and E). The small areas of hemorrhage are shown as ovoid black areas with white halo due to magnetic susceptibility (arrows).

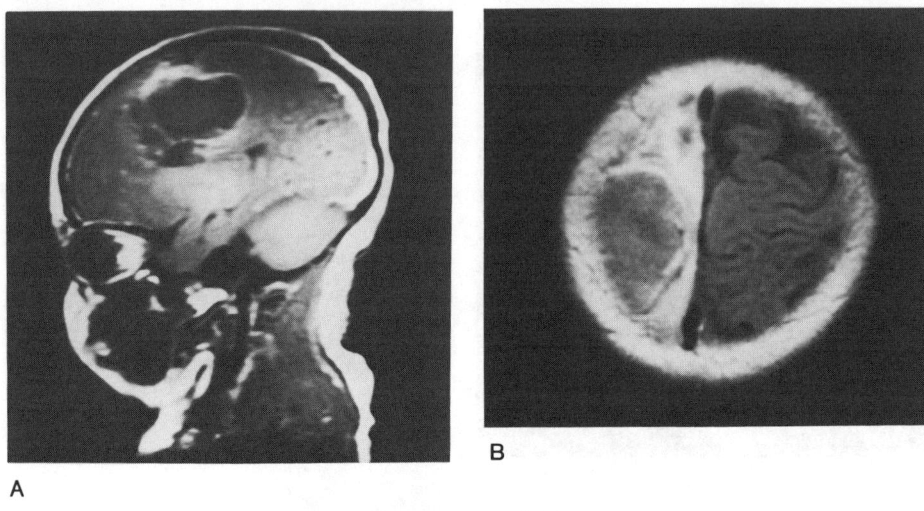

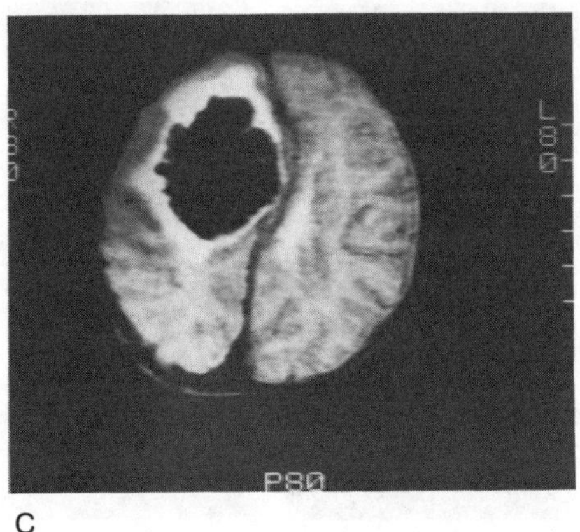

Figure 4.7 Acute intraparenchymal hematoma. (A) Sagittal T_1 weighted MR shows large acute intraparenchymal hematoma as oval black area with thin white rim. Note subdural hematoma at vertex shown as crescent-shaped white area. (B) Axial T_1 weighted MR shows oval hematoma on the right oval gray area surrounded by thin white rim. (C) Axial T_2 weighted MR shows acute intraparenchymal hematoma as oval black area surrounded by white area representing edema.

cially if time has passed, because there is evolutionary change from deoxyhemoglobin to methemoglobin and later to hemosiderin [2]. For example, CT detection of subarachnoid hemorrhage (SAH) is better seen acutely and is seen less well with the passage of time. With MR, the SAH may not be seen acutely but may be seen later as evolutionary changes take place [18,19].

MR is much more sensitive than CT in the detection of edema. The areas of perifocal edema associated with contusion or hematoma appear to be more

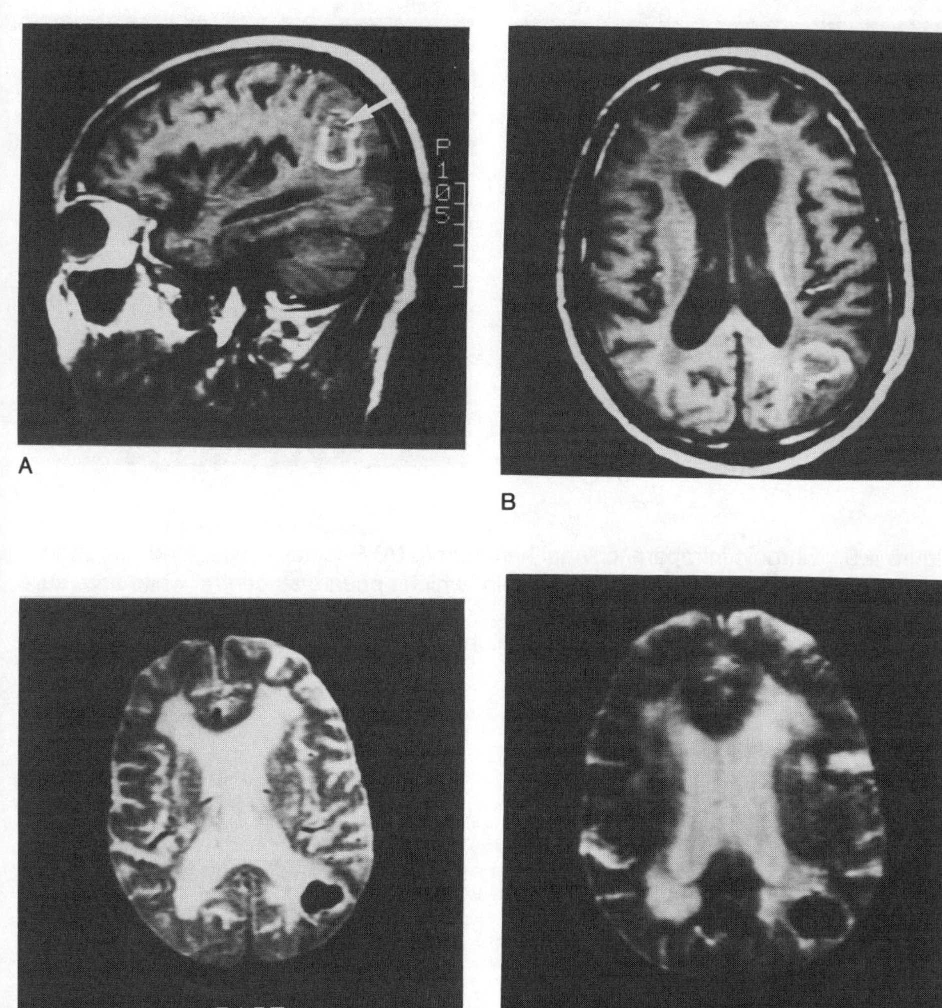

Figure 4.8 Subacute intraparenchymal hematoma. (A) Sagittal T_1 weighted MR shows oval subacute intraparenchymal hematoma in left parietal area (arrow) with thick white rim indicating methemoglobin formation. (B) Axial T_1 weighted MR demonstrating the hematoma. (C) Axial T_2 weighted MR shows the central portion of the hematoma as black (deoxyhemoglobin) with white rim (methemoglobin). (D) Axial "fast scan" using gradient-recalled techniques. The black center of the hematoma appears somewhat larger due to "magnetic susceptibility."

extensive and persist longer than as indicated by CT [1]. Small areas of "nonhemorrhagic contusion" that may not be detectable by CT may be visualized by MR on T_2 weighted sequences, probably because the edema is detected (Figures 4.11 and 4.12) [8,15,16].

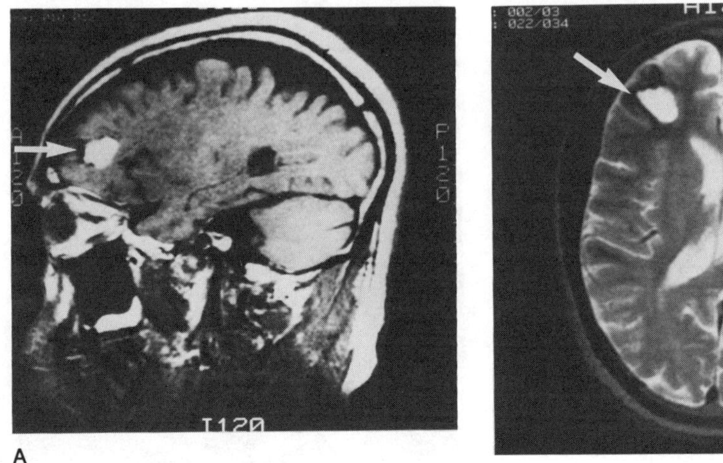

Figure 4.9　Chronic intraparenchymal hematoma. (A) Sagittal T_1 weighted MR shows conversion of hematoma to methemoglobin, which appears as central white area surrounded by black rim composed of hemosiderin (arrow). (B) Axial T_2 weighted MR shows white area composed of methemoglobin, with black rim of hemosiderin (arrow).

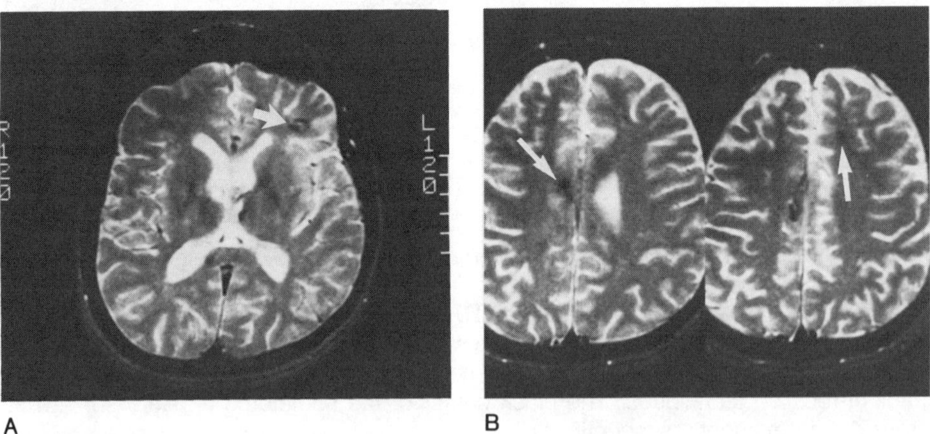

Figure 4.10　Old hemorrhagic contusions. Axial T_2 weighted MR images show black areas of old hemorrhagic contusion with hemosiderin formation: (A) in the left frontal area (arrow), and (B) in the right frontal-parietal vertex and left centrum semiovale (arrows). These contusions were two years old based on clinical history.

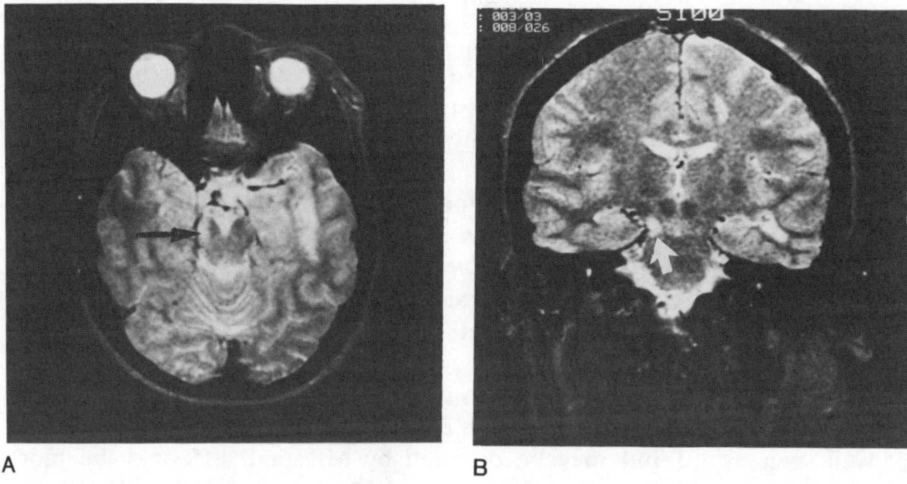

Figure 4.11　Brain stem contusion. (A) Axial T$_2$ weighted MR shows white-appearing area of increased signal intensity representing contusion in the right cerebral peduncle. (B) Coronal T$_2$ weighted MR confirms location in right cerebral peduncle (arrow). This lesion was seen in a patient with unexplained hemiparesis following trauma, and was not detected by CT.

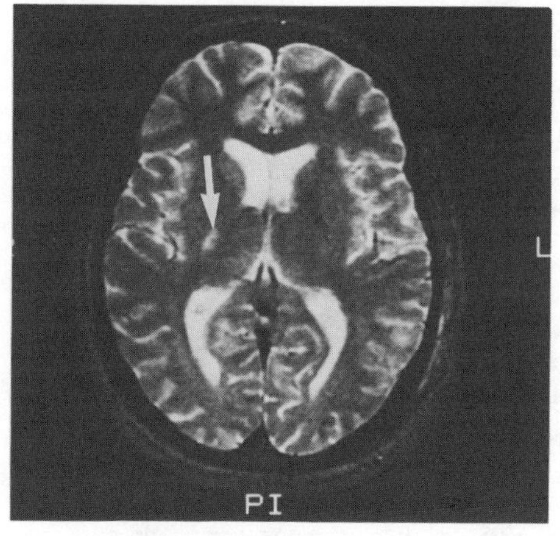

Figure 4.12　Shearing injury. Axial T$_2$ weighted MR shows injuries (arrow) in the posterior limb of the right internal capsule. This is demonstrated by MR primarily because of the associated edema, and this lesion was not detected by CT.

It is important to detect lesions in the deep white matter of frontal and temporal lobes, corpus callosum, corona radiata, and brain stem that may be associated with coma and poor prognosis [20,21]. These lesions may not be detected with CT, and yet may be defined by MR (Figure 4.6). This includes the posttraumatic diffuse axonal injury produced by shearing forces in the white matter at the moment of impact, now recognized as a cause of severe neuropsychological deficit [6,9,14–16,21–23]. Large intraparenchymal hematomas can be detected by either modality. Some medical centers are fairly aggressive in draining these hematomas if they cause pressure on vital structures. Examples would be in the cerebellum where pressure is exerted on the brain stem, or in herniation syndromes related to focal hematomas.

Of particular importance may be the superiority of MR in detecting lesions in the area of the brain stem and temporal lobes as compared with CT. The pons, and portions of the midbrain and medial temporal lobes, are frequently obscured by artifact on CT scans. However, one must be aware of a number of artifacts in these same areas that also occur in MR (most of which are related to cerebrospinal fluid flow or arterial pulsations). These artifacts should not be mistaken for pathology [14,17].

Other long-term sequelae of brain trauma, such as posttraumatic atrophy or hydrocephalus, can be detected with either modality. However, "gliosis" is not well seen by CT but may be detected by MR, and MR may be more sensitive in the early detection of posttraumatic infarction. Differentiation of gliosis from focal edema caused by contusion or infarction must generally be made with the help of clinical history because their MR appearance is not specific [1]. In the follow-up of trauma patients, the insertion of metallic pressure-monitoring devices or ventriculostomy tubes with metallic parts will have a more profound detrimental effect on MR images than on CT. Abnormalities in the diploic space of the calvarium, such as posttraumatic osteomyelitis, may be demonstrated better by MR than by CT [9]. Postconcussion syndrome may not show any definite abnormality on MR or CT.

CT may remain the modality generally used for screening acute brain trauma at present, because most surgically treatable abnormalities are well detected by CT. However, MR has certain advantages, particularly in the long-term follow-up and prognosis of brain injuries. As time passes, MR is likely to be used more and more for the initial evaluation as well as the follow-up of brain injury.

REFERENCES

1. Bradley WG. Pathophysiologic correlates of signal alteration. In: Brant-Zawadski M, Norman D, eds. Magnetic resonance imaging of the central nervous system. New York: Raven Press, 1986;23–42.
2. Gomori JM, Grossman RI, Goldberg HI, Zimmerman RA, Bilaniuk LT. Intracranial hematomas: Imaging by high-field MR. Radiology 1985;157(1):87-89.
3. Edelman RR, Johnson K, Buxton R, et al: MR of hemorrhage: A new approach. AJNR 1986;7:751–56.
4. McArdle CB, Nicholas DA, Richardson CJ: Monitoring of the newborn undergoing MR imaging: Technical considerations. Radiology 1986;159:223–26.
5. Kelly WM, Paglen PG, Pearson JA, San Diego AG, Soloman MA. Ferromagnetism of intraocular foreign body causes unilateral blindness after MR study. AJNR 1986;7:243–45.

6. Gentry LR, Godersky JC, Thompson B, Dunn VD: Prospective comparative study of intermediate-field MR and CT in the evaluation of closed head trauma. AJNR 1988;9:91–100.

7. Moon KL, Brant-Zawadzki M, Pitts LH, Mills CM. Nuclear magnetic resonance imaging of CT-isodense subdural hematomas. AJNR 1984;5:319–22.

8. Snow RB, Zimmerman RD, Gandy SE, Deck MD. Comparison of magnetic resonance imaging and computed tomography in the evaluation of head injury. Neurosurgery 1986;18(1):45–52.

9. Han JS, Kaufman B, Alfidi RJ, Yeung HN, Benson JE, Haaga JR, El Yousef SJ, Clampitt ME, Bonstelle CT, Huss R. Head trauma evaluated by magnetic resonance and computed tomography: A comparison. Radiology 1984;150:71–77.

10. Sipponen JT, Sipponen RE, Sivula A: Chronic subdural hematoma: Demonstration by magnetic resonance. Radiology 1984;150:79–85.

11. Han JS, Benson JE, Kaufman B, Rekate HL, Alfidi RJ, Huss RG, Sacco D, Yoon YS, Morrison SC. MR imaging of pediatric cerebral abnormalities. J Comput Assist Tomogr 1985;9(1):103–14.

12. Zimmerman RA, Bilaniuk LT, Hackney DB, Goldberg HI, Grossman RI. Paranasal sinus hemorrhage: Evaluation with MR imaging. Radiology 1987;162:499–503.

13. McArdle CB, Amparo EG, Mirfakhraee M. MR imaging of orbital blow-out fractures. J Comput Assist Tomogr 1986;10(1):116–19.

14. Gentry LR, Godersky JC, Thompson B. MR imaging of head trauma: Review of the distribution and radiopathologic features of traumatic lesions. AJNR 1988;9:101–10.

15. Hesselink JR, Dowd CF, Healy ME, Hajek P, Baker LL, Luerssen TG. MR imaging of the brain contusions: A comparative study with CT. AJNR 1988;9:269–78.

16. Zimmerman RA, Bilaniuk LT, Hackney DB, Goldberg HI, Grossman RI. Head injury: Early results of comparing CT and high-field MR. AJR 1986;147:1215–22.

17. Kelley WM: Image artifacts and technical limitations. In: Brant-Zawadski M, Norman D, eds. Magnetic resonance imaging of the central nervous system, New York: Raven Press, 1986;43–82.

18. Chakeres DW, Bryan RN. Acute subarachnoid hemorrhage: In vitro comparison of magnetic resonance and computed tomography. AJNR 1986;7:223–28.

19. Bradley WG, Schmidt PG. Effect of methemoglobin formation on the MR appearance of subarachnoid hemorrhage. Radiology 1985;156:99–103.

20. Norman D. Vascular disease: Hemorrhage. In: Brant-Zawadski M, Norman D, eds. Magnetic resonance imaging of the central nervous system. New York: Raven Press, 1986;209–34.

21. Jenkins A, Teasdale G, Handley MDM, Macpherson P, Rowan JO. Brain lesions detected by magnetic resonance imaging in mild and severe head injuries. Lancet 1986;2(8504):445–46.

22. Levin HS, Handel SF, Goldman AM, Eisenberg HM, Guinto FC Jr. Magnetic resonance imaging after "diffuse" nonmissile head injury. A neurobehavioral study. Arch Neurol 1985;42:963–68.

23. Lipper MH, Kishore PRS, Enas GG, Domingues da Silva AA, Choi SC, Becker DP. Computed tomography in the prediction of outcome in head injury. AJNR 1985;6:7–10.

SUGGESTED READING

Bilaniuk LT, Zimmerman PA, Wehrli FW, Goldberg HI, Grossman RI, Bottomley PA, Edelstein WA, Glover GH, MacFall JR, Redington RW, Kressel HY. Cerebral magnetic resonance: Comparison of high and low field strength imaging. Radiology 1984; 153:409–14.

Young IR, Bydder GM, Hall AS, Steiner RE, Worthington BS, Hawkes RC, Holland GN, Moore WS. Extracerebral collections: Recognition by NMR imaging. AJNR 1983;4:883-34.

Chapter 5

New Technology in Intracranial Dynamics Following Head Injury

Steven J. Allen

During the past twenty years, our understanding of the pathophysiology of acute head injury has markedly increased. This insight has been accompanied by an approach typified by the patient's admission to an intensive care unit, identification and timely evacuation of hematomas, cardiopulmonary support, and treatment of intercranial hypertension. However, the incidence of unsatisfactory outcome continues to be high. Improvements in therapy are currently limited by the relatively crude monitors we have for determining the development of adverse conditions in the injured brain. Thus, therapeutic interventions tend to be empirical, and to be made relatively late in the disease process. If we are to positively affect the course of acute head injury further, we will need to monitor the injured brain more specifically to titrate therapy to the particular pathophysiologic process. This chapter reviews current efforts at improving standard monitors and discusses new technology and its potential impact on patient care.

INTRACRANIAL PRESSURE

Since the original clinical descriptions of intracranial pressure (ICP) [1,2], its impact on the outcome of acutely head-injured patients has attracted much attention. Clinical studies have correlated the severity of intracranial hypertension with mortality and have suggested that lowering increased ICP improves outcome [3,4]. Although some patients with elevated ICP, such as those with pseudotumor cerebri, appear to suffer no acute neurologic deterioration, the same does not hold for patients with acute head injuries. Intracranial hypertension may result in ischemia by compression of the local vasculature already damaged from injury, or may exacerbate trauma-induced distortions of cerebral architecture, leading to further ischemia, herniation, or both. Clinical experience, laboratory research, and theoretical considerations compel the conclusion that the control of intracranial hypertension is a major clinical goal in patients with acute head injuries.

The intracranial vault contains the cerebral blood volume, the cerebrospinal fluid, and the brain parenchyma. ICP may be elevated by an increase in any of these compartments. The cerebral blood volume may be elevated by hypercarbia, hypoxia, hypertension, seizures, elevated jugular venous pressure, and trauma-induced cerebral hyperemia. The brain parenchyma volume may be increased by the development of edema. The cerebrospinal fluid compartment may increase due to obstruction of the absorption pathways leading to hydrocephalus. Rather than a stereotypic approach to all elevations of ICP, the prevention and management of intercranial hypertension should be aimed at the particular cause.

The management of ICP requires a reliable method of measurement. Currently, the vast majority of ICP monitors in clinical use are of two types. Ventriculostomy requires the insertion of a fluid-filled tube into a frontal horn of one of the lateral ventricles. The advantages of this system are that the pressure recording is reliable and cerebrospinal fluid can be drained as needed. Recently, a fiberoptic, transducer-tipped ventricular catheter has been introduced into clinical use that offers superior waveform fidelity. The other method of monitoring ICP involves transducing the pressure just above the cortex by means of fluid-filled or transducer-tipped bolts. Technically, these devices are more easily placed, but their reliability has been questioned [5].

A major problem with ICP monitors is that they are invasive. Placement is not a benign procedure. Reported complications include hemorrhage, infection, and further neuronal loss. One attempt to reduce the morbidity of ICP monitoring has led to the development of a telemetry ICP monitor. The Rotterdam Teletransducer can be implanted in the skull and enclosed completely under the skin to measure epidural pressure. Initial clinical experience in patients with acute severe head injury is promising [6].

Recognition of the elasticity of the skull has led to another prototypic noninvasive ICP monitor. Pitlyk et al placed a set of strain gauges on the center of Gardner-Wells tongs (commonly used for spinal traction). They found that their device could detect a change as small as 2 mm Hg in the ICP in dogs. Furthermore, the device could even pick up the rhythmic changes in the bitemporal diameter of the skull induced by cardiac cycle. A major drawback of this technique is that the device cannot be zeroed [7].

Niroscopy (near infrared optical spectroscopy) has been developed as a potential bedside technique to monitor the adverse effects of increased ICP. This method measures the absorbance peaks for hemoglobin, cytochrome a,a3, and oxyhemoglobin. Cytochrome a,a3 is the terminal member in the mitochondrial electron transport chain that accounts for more than 90% of cellular oxygen use in aerobic metabolism. Thus, the relative redox state of this critical molecule can be continuously ascertained. Furthermore, by suitable algorithms, the relative changes in cerebral hemoglobin saturation and blood volume can be determined. In animal studies, increases in ICP have been associated with reduction of both cytochrome a,a3 and oxyhemoglobin [8]. Limited clinical studies have included preterm infants and anesthetized patients [9,10]. There are two hurdles to overcome in the future. First, unless a patient can be monitored before injury, no baseline can be determined. That is, the device gives only a relative value of the intracranial variables. Second, it is not clear at what level of a,a3 reduction the cerebral ischemia develops. The device can monitor trends but is not able to identify when a truly adverse situation has arisen.

Regardless of how ICP is measured, a fundamental problem exists with basing therapy on the ICP value. We need to know if some or all of the brain is compromised and, if so, for what reason. We then need to have an intervention that may correct the problem, and the ability to quickly ascertain whether an improvement has been achieved. Intracranial hypertension in itself does not necessarily correlate with cerebral ischemia. More certainly, a low ICP does not guarantee that all is well. Future management of acute head injuries must use better markers of intracranial metabolism.

For most determinations of regional cerebral blood flow (CBF) in the head-injured population, xenon 133 has been administered, with detection by external counters [11]. This technique allows for the determination of regional CBF only in those areas of the brain near the detectors. No information is given concerning deeper areas of the brain, and only global measurements of metabolism can be obtained.

ANATOMIC IMAGING

For a number of conditions occurring in the patient with acute head injury, surgery is the appropriate intervention. Key to the treatment of these lesions is the ability to promptly and reliably identify the presence of such conditions. During the past 15 years, CT of the brain has replaced carotid angiography and revolutionized the imaging of intracranial masses. However, the quality of CT scans is adversely affected by bone. Thus, the posterior fossa, being surrounded by the petrous ridges, is often difficult to visualize. Furthermore, CT distinguishes structure solely by the x-ray absorption of the underlying tissue. Thus, masses, such as some hematomas, can appear isodense with parenchyma and may not be well defined by CT.

The clinical introduction of magnetic resonance imaging (MR) appears to offer a technical improvement in imaging compared with conventional CT. Current MR spatially identifies and relatively quantifies the concentration of hydrogen nuclei (each of which consists of a single proton). These nuclei, and others of a certain spin, act as magnets. When placed in a strong magnetic field, these nuclei tend to become aligned with the magnetic field. They do not completely line up; rather, they "wobble" (precess) around the magnetic field at a reproducible frequency (resonance) called the Lamor frequency. If an electromagnetic signal of this same Lamor frequency is directed at these nuclei perpendicular to the magnetic field, the nuclei will absorb some of the energy. When the electromagnetic signal is turned off, the nuclei will release the absorbed energy at an intensity relative to the number of nuclei present. The decay of this release of energy can be used to create images. Because the hydrogen content of bone is relatively low, MR images of the posterior fossa are excellent. In one study, 35 patients with acute brain injury underwent both CT and MR. MR was superior in imaging 23 of 41 extracerebral fluid collections and in visualizing nonhemorrhagic contusions in 15 of 21 lesions [12]. However, the additional information obtained with MR did not change the surgical management of any patient. Furthermore, MR was not as good as CT in identifying acute subarachnoid hemorrhage or acute parenchymal hemorrhage. MR uses a powerful magnet that limits the kinds of material that may be near the scanner. Because patients often have life-sustaining apparatus attached to them at the time of the scan, MR scanning poses certain logistical problems.

MR and CT are not portable. Many patients who require imaging are extremely sick, and being transported to the radiology department is not always in their best interest. Ultrasound imaging is portable but does not penetrate bone. Reports on the use of ultrasound imaging in patients with craniectomy defects have prompted some clinicians to modify the burr hole made for the ICP monitor so that the portable ultrasound probe can be used [13]. Because rapid identification of intracranial hematomas is crucial to optimal patient outcome, we may see cerebral ultrasonography performed at the bedside in the emergency department and intensive care unit.

METABOLIC MONITORING

Standard management for acute head injury is unusual in that the first line of therapy is to reduce blood flow to the injured organ. Empiric hyperventilation is instituted without regard to whether the CBF will be decreased too much. Indeed, Obrist et al found that, in the presence of normocarbia and normotension, almost half the head-injured patients studied had relative cerebral hyperemia that correlated with the presence of intercranial hypertension [11]. In the patients with hyperemia, CBF was not coupled to the underlying cerebral oxygen consumption ($CMRO_2$). These patients typically retained CO_2 responsiveness and responded well to hyperventilation. The rest of the patients had lower CBF values that appeared coupled to the $CMRO_2$. In some of these patients, these investigators found that routine hyperventilation could lead to reductions in CBF sufficient to suggest ischemia. CBF and $CMRO_2$ can be measured in patients but are still largely investigational. However, the absolute values of CBF and $CMRO_2$ are not necessary. To diagnose whether relative hyperemia or hypoperfusion exists, only a measurement of the relationship of $CMRO_2$ to CBF is needed. The Fick equation for the brain is:

$$CMRO_2 = CBF \times AJDO_2, \tag{1}$$

where $AJDO_2$ is the arterial jugular venous oxygen content difference. Rearranging the equation,

$$CMRO_2/CBF = AJDO_2. \tag{2}$$

$AJDO_2$ represents the ratio of $CMRO_2$ to a measure of cerebral oxygen delivery (CBF). $AJDO_2$ can be determined by the standard laboratory measurement of hemoglobin concentration and saturation of arterial and jugular venous blood. The latter is obtained by placing a catheter into the superior portion of the jugular bulb via a retrograde insertion in an internal jugular vein. The normal value for $AJDO_2$ is 6.3 ± 1.2 ml of oxygen per 100 ml of blood. When $AJDO_2$ is elevated, CBF is relatively low for $CMRO_2$, implying that the brain is having to extract more oxygen from the blood delivered. Conversely, a low $AJDO_2$ value suggests relative hyperemia. Thus, in a patient with intracranial hypertension, a low $AJDO_2$ value indicates further hyperventilation to reduce the CBF and the ICP. However, an elevated $AJDO_2$ implies that the CBF should not be lowered further. Rather, a treatment should be used that lowers ICP but increases CBF. Mannitol has been shown to have these characteristics. This approach of titrating $PaCO_2$ and mannitol to normalize the $AJDO_2$ allows for therapy tailored to the patient's particular CBF response to head trauma. We have had experience with a system of continuous $AJDO_2$ monitoring using indwelling oximetry catheters [13]. This system allows for immediate bedside response to changes in the patient's global CBF and metabolism. The major disadvantage is that the measurement is only a global one. Local areas of mismatch between flow and metabolism may be missed completely. This is especially true for the posterior fossa, which contributes a fraction to the total cerebral venous outflow but whose function is extremely critical.

Positron emission tomography (PET) offers the opportunity in the near future to routinely monitor regional flow and metabolism in cerebral disease. As opposed to anatomic imaging techniques, such as CT, that offer only structural information, PET scanning provides a three-dimensional reconstruction of CBF and metabolic function. The scans are obtained by administering positron-emitting isotopes to patients. These positrons travel a short distance and annihilate with an electron to give rise to two photons that travel in opposite directions. PET scanners consist of an array of photon detectors that are designed to record a signal only when opposing detectors are simultaneously struck by photons. By using various labeled compounds, regional values for cerebral pH, cerebral blood volume, CBF, $CMRO_2$, glucose metabolism, and blood-brain barrier permeability can be determined. A preliminary report of three head-injured patients was made by Langfitt et al that included CT, MR, PET, and xenon-133 CBF determinations [14]. This study demonstrated that the decrease in glucose metabolism found by PET was more extensive than that of structural injury shown by CT or MR. A disadvantage of PET is that, due to the short half-lives of the radiopharmaceuticals, there must be a cyclotron in the vicinity of the scanner. Second, the glucose determination requires 45 minutes for the scan and a 9-hour wait before the scan can be repeated. Finally, knowing the relative or even absolute numbers of flow, volume, or even metabolism, does not tell us whether an adverse situation is present. We still need some indicator of cellular integrity. A step in that direction might be the use of misonidazole compounds that bind preferentially to hypoxic cells [15]. These compounds can be radiolabled and could act as regional markers of inadequate blood supply.

Nuclear magnetic resonance (NMR) spectroscopy is in its infancy, but it may ultimately provide basic answers in the management of acute head injuries. The techniques above may, at best, be able to identify regions of relatively low CBF to cerebral metabolism. However, they cannot determine whether ischemia is present. Oxygen is carried by hemoglobin to the capillaries, where it is released and diffuses into cells. The mitochondria take up oxygen and reduce it to form water and produce adenosine triphosphate (ATP) and phosphocreatine, which act as energy sources. The energy is released when inorganic phosphate is catalyzed from the molecule. As oxygen delivery decreases, production of ATP by the mitochondria also begins to decrease. Phosphocreatine is used as an energy store to help maintain levels of ATP. Cellular hypoxia results in a decline in the phosphocreatine level and an increase in inorganic phosphate. NMR spectroscopy can measure the relative intracellular concentration of these various phosphorous-containing compounds. Thus, this technique can determine when an area has been rendered ischemic by therapy or disease process. Hilberman et al used NMR spectroscopy to measure the effect of hypoxemia on dog brains. They found that, when the arterial oxygen tension was less than 30 mm Hg, phosphocreatine levels and inorganic phosphate levels rose [16]. However, the ability to apply NMR spectroscopy throughout the brain is many years away, because spatial localization is a major problem.

Another approach to monitoring the central nervous system is to examine the special function of neuronal cells, that is, their electrical activity. The standard monitor of neuronal function is the neurologic exam. However, in patients who are deeply comatose or who are under the influence of such therapeutic agents as muscle relaxants and barbiturates, the neurologic exam is not helpful in assessing the integrity of the nervous system. Electrophysiologic monitoring has been developed that is useful in these situations and can be accomplished in two basic ways. First, spontaneous electrical activity (electroencephalography [EEG]) can be monitored by placing electrodes around the scalp. The EEG is difficult to interpret without special training, and the amount of data generated makes it impractical for continuous monitoring. The compressed spectral array (CSA) produces more manageable information by waveform analysis and may have a place in the treatment of head-injured patients, but its influence on patient management has yet to be determined. Monitoring of sensory evoked potentials is another neurophysiologic technique that attempts to determine the functional integrity of the central nervous system. If a sensory stimulus is applied at a peripheral afferent sensory nerve, the arrival of that impulse in the appropriate part of the brain can be detected by scalp electrodes after appropriate signal filtering and averaging have been performed. Somatosensory, auditory, and visual afferent pathways have been characterized in a number of clinical situations. Impairment of neuronal integrity can be deduced by both the time the impulse takes to get to the brain and the particular pattern of response. Most of the experience with sensory evoked potentials has been obtained in the operating room. The place of this type of monitoring has yet to be ascertained, but it appears promising as an on-line technique in the intensive care unit.

SUMMARY

A major direction in monitoring techniques is toward the detection of regional ischemia. However, identifying mismatches of regional blood flow to metabolism will be of benefit only if therapy to correct these focal problems is available. There is some evidence that certain pharmacologic interventions, such as barbiturates [17], calcium entry blockers [18], or mannitol [19] may cause a redistribution of blood flow to these ischemic areas. However, there is little proof that such redistribution improves outcome.

Because of the explosion of technology now available to study patients, we need to better define our goals. Technology should be guided in two directions. First, we should determine when to intervene, and what interventions are most appropriate. As with cerebral vascular accidents and spinal cord injury studies, the timing of the interventions may be more important than the actual agent. Once the injury pattern has been initiated, the outcome may be set. Second, society must manage its resources efficiently. We should set as a goal the identification of those patients for whom an unsatisfactory outcome is highly probable regardless of management. This will require rigorous collection of data on patients who undergo standardized therapy. Only in this fashion can we assure ourselves that we are making a difference in the clinical management of these head-injured patients.

REFERENCES

1. Guillaume J, Janny P. Manometrie intracranienne continue: Interêt de la method et premiers resultats. Rev Neurol 1951;84:131–42.
2. Lundberg N. Continuous recording and control of ventricular fluid pressure in neurosurgical practice. Acta Psychiatr Neurol Scand 1960;36(Suppl 149):1–193.
3. Miller JD, Becker DP, Ward JD, Sullivan HG, Adams WE, Rosner MJ. Significance of intracranial hypertension in severe head injury. J Neurosurg 1977;47:503–16.
4. Saul TG, Ducker TB. Effect of intracranial pressure monitoring and aggressive treatment on mortality in severe head injury. J Neurosurg 1982;56:498–503.
5. Miller JD, Bobo H, Kapp JP. Inaccurate pressure readings for subarachnoid bolts. Neurosurgery 1986;19(2):253–55.

6. Maas AIR, de Jong DA. The Rotterdam teletransducer: State of the device. Acta Neurochir 1986;79:5–12.
7. Pitlyk PJ, Piantanida TP, Ploeger DW. Noninvasive intracranial pressure monitoring. Neurosurgery 1985;17(4):581–84.
8. Cairns CB, Fillipo D, Proctor HJ. A noninvasive method for monitoring the effects of increased intracranial pressure with near infrared spectrophotometry. Surg Gynecol Obstet 1985;161:145–48.
9 Brazy JE, Lewis DV, Mitnick MH, van der Vleit FFJ. Noninvasive monitoring of cerebral oxygenation in preterm infants: Preliminary observations. Pediatrics 1985; 75(2):217–25.
10. Macek C. Device gauges anesthetized patient's brain O_2. JAMA 1982;248(17):2086–87.
11. Obrist WD, Langfitt TW, Jaggi JL, Cruz J, Gennarelli TA. Cerebral blood flow and metabolism in comatose patients with acute head injury. J Neurosurg 1984;61:241–53.
12. Snow RB, Zimmerman RD, Gandy SE, Deck MDF. Comparison of magnetic resonance imaging and computed tomography in the evaluation of head injury. Neurosurgery 1986;18(1):45–52.
13. Ostrop R, Bejar R, Marshall L. Real-time ultrasonography: Evaluation of the craniectomized, brain-injured patient. Neurosurgery 1984;12:225–27.
14. Langfitt TW, Obrist WD, Alavi A, Grossman RI, Zimmerman R, Jaggi J, Uzzell B, Reivich M, Patton DR. Computerized tomography, magnetic resonance imaging, and positron emission tomography in the study of brain trauma. J Neurosurg 1986;64:760–67.
15. Grunbaum Z, Freauff SJ, Krohn KA, Wilbur DS, Magee S, Rasey JS. Synthesis and characterization of congeners of misonidazole for imaging hypoxia. J Nucl Med 1987;28:68–75.
16. Hilberman M, Subramanian VH, Haselgrove J, Cone JB, Egan JW, Gyulai L, Chance B. In vivo time-resolved brain phosphorus nuclear magnetic resonance. J Cereb Blood Flow Metab 1984;4:334–42.
17. Ochiai C, Asano T, Takakura K, Fukda T, Horizoe H, Morimoto Y. Mechanism of cerebral protection by pentobarbital and nizofenone correlated with the course of local cerebral blood flow changes. Stroke 1982;13(6):788–96.
18. Harris RJ, Branston NM, Symon L, Bayhan M, Watson A. The effects of a calcium antagonist, nimodipine upon physiological responses of the cerebral vasculature and its possible influence upon focal cerebral ischemia. Stroke 1982;13(6):759–66.
19. Ravussin P, Archer DP, Tyler JL, Meyer E, Abou-Madi M, Diksic M, Yamamoto L, Trop D. Effects of rapid mannitol infusion on cerebral blood volume. A positron emission tomographic study in dogs and man. J Neurosurg 1986;64:104–13.
20. Cruz J, Allen SJ, Miner ME. Hypoxic insults in acute brain injury. Crit Care Med 1985;13:284.

Chapter 6

The Treatment of Severely Brain-Injured Patients with Hyperbaric Oxygen

Gaylan L. Rockswold
David C. Anderson
Sandra E. Ford

The history of hyperbaric oxygen (HBO) for the treatment of brain injury is long and somewhat checkered. A survey of published material suggests that this modality has been underutilized as a clinical tool in the treatment of traumatic cerebral edema. In 1983 a clinical trial was begun at Hennepin County Medical Center to learn which severely head-injured patients, if any, benefit from HBO, and in what ways they benefit.

REVIEW OF EXPERIMENTAL AND CLINICAL STUDIES

HBO increases the amount of oxygen dissolved in the plasma many times, depending on the absolute pressure used. At 2 atmospheres absolute (ATA), it increases arterial oxygen tension to between 1,000 and 1,250 mm Hg [1] and decreases cerebral blood flow (CBF) by approximately 22% [2–6]. The reduction in CBF may be due to cerebral vasoconstriction; several investigators have demonstrated that it is *not* dependent on hypocarbia [7–9]. When cerebral autoregulation is lost, CBF no longer decreases with the administration of HBO [10,11].

Corresponding with the reduction in CBF secondary to cerebral vasoconstriction, there is experimental and clinical evidence that reduction in the intracranial pressure (ICP) occurs. Miller et al demonstrated in several experimental studies that ICP decreases by about one-third of the control value with the application of HBO [1,9]. Both cold lesions of the cerebral cortex and extradural balloons were used in these experiments. Sukoff and Ragatz reported on a series of 50 patients with traumatic cerebral edema who were treated with HBO [12]. In 10 of these, ICP was systematically monitored. The ICPs during HBO were consistently lower than those before HBO ($P < 0.001$), and the reductions were sustained for 2 to 4 hours after HBO in most cases. Other investigators have not reported such a consistent response. Hayakawa et al measured cerebral spinal fluid pressure via a needle inserted in the cisterna magna in 26 dogs [13]. They found a consistent decrease in pressure during the first 20 to 30 minutes of HBO but then a tendency for the pressures to return toward baseline. However, these animals were treated at 3 ATA, and Miller found ICP reduction relatively resistant at pressures greater than 2 ATA [1]. Hayakawa et al also studied the changes in cerebral spinal fluid pressure with HBO in 13 patients suffering acute cerebral damage [13]. In nine of these patients who had sustained closed-head injury, pressure decreased at the beginning of HBO and reverted rapidly with decompression. There was a tendency to some rebound after cessation of treatment.

Holbach et al studied glucose metabolism in 23 patients who had acute cerebral injuries [14]. While the patients breathed air and oxygen at normobaric pressure and then again at 1.5 and 2.0 ATA, the cerebral arteriovenous differences for oxygen, glucose, lactate, pyruvate, blood gas pressures, and pH values were measured. There was a distinctly increased cerebral glycolysis while patients breathed air, indicating insufficient oxygen delivery to the brain. The change from breathing air to oxygen resulted in a distinct inhibition of cerebral glycolysis, indicating improved cerebral oxygenation and energy production. At an inspiratory oxygen pressure of 1.5 ATA, cerebral glucose metabolism was nearly balanced, indicating adequate cerebral oxygenation and energy formation. A further increase in inspiratory oxygen pressure to 2.0 ATA increased cerebral glycolysis considerably. This was assumed to be due to cerebral oxygen poisoning resulting in disturbed oxidative energy formation. Artu et al studied similar parameters in brain-injured patients treated with HBO at 2.5 ATA [15]. His results were less consistent and less suggestive that HBO was beneficial in cerebral glucose metabolism. However, the study of Holbach et al suggests that 2.5 ATA is an excessive pressure for ideal glucose metabolism [14].

The causes of high mortality and morbidity in severe brain injury are multifaceted. The brain's response to the particular injury is proportional to the severity. Vasogenic edema may be focal or diffuse throughout the brain, leading to elevated ICP [16]. Hypoxia and hypercarbia can lead to cerebral vasodilatation, elevated CBF, and further cerebral edema. A vicious cycle can occur with loss of autoregulation [17]. Focal or diffuse ischemia can result from brain shifts occluding or partially occluding the anterior and posterior cerebral arteries, from traction on central perforating arteries to the brain stem, or from failure of arterial pressure to maintain adequate perfusion pressures [18,19]. Glucose metabolism appears to decrease in severe brain injury even if CBF has increased [20]. It seemed useful to investigate a treatment that might affect ICP by (1) reducing CBF by vasoconstriction, and (2) simultaneously supplying oxygen at a level that would provide optimum cerebral glucose aerobic metabolism.

Indeed, there are a number of experimental and clinical studies suggesting that HBO reduces the mortality and morbidity caused by cerebral edema. Sukoff et al studied the protective effect of HBO in experimental cerebral edema in 44 dogs [21]. Sperl et al placed dry sterilized psyllium seed into the white matter to produce local cerebral edema by a slowly expanding intracranial space-occupying lesion [22]. Within 24 hours of psyllium seed implantation in 32 dogs, HBO was instituted at 3.0 ATA for 45 minutes every 8 hours; survival was studied. Beginning on day 2 after seed implantation, the control animals showed a progressive downhill course characterized by hemiparesis and a decreased level of consciousness. Death occurred in 83% by day 8. In the HBO group, progressive neurologic deterioration was interrupted. By day 8, surviving treated animals were neurologically normal except for mild contralateral weakness; mortality was 27%. Analyses of these data reveal statistically significant differences in outcome. Cisternal punctures in the control animals showed a steady elevation of pressure on successive days, whereas cisternal punctures in the HBO-treated animals performed immediately before and after a treatment session demonstrated a consistent drop in pressure.

In a second article, Sukoff et al described the placement of an extradural balloon in the left frontoparietal area [23]. Animals were observed during a one-week recovery period; those showing neurologic or systemic deficits were excluded from the study. On day 8 postoperation, balloons were inflated with 5 cm³ of 50% Hypaque solution over 2 minutes in one group of dogs and over 10 minutes in another. HBO treatment was carried out as described above, except that it began immediately following balloon inflation. In the 22 dogs in whom balloon inflation occurred over 10 minutes, 12 served as controls. All animals showed a progressive deterioration in level of consciousness with contralateral hemiparesis and ipsilateral pupillary dilation by the time the balloon expansion was completed. Although varying degrees of spontaneous improvement occurred in the control group, the mortality was ultimately 100% by day four postinflation. In the 10 animals treated by intermittent exposure to HBO immediately after balloon inflation, mortality was 50%. Survivors were normal by day 6 postinflation. Analysis of these data reveals a highly significant statistical difference in outcome. HBO also provided protection to the animals during rapid (2 minutes) inflation of the balloon. Four control dogs became rapidly comatose and decerebrate and died within 30 minutes to 12 hours. In another four animals, balloons were also inflated over 2 minutes while the animals were breathing 100% oxygen at 3 ATA. Evidence of some discomfort and mild contralateral weakness was seen during balloon inflation. All remained in stable condition until they were killed 12 hours later. A similar study was performed by Moody et al using an extradural balloon in dogs [24]. The 95% mortality rate in the control group was reduced to 50% by treatment with 100% oxygen at 2 ATA for 4 hours following balloon decompression. Quality of survival was good among dogs in the treated group.

Several articles describe the clinical use of HBO in the treatment of severe cerebral injuries. Mogami et al reported on the use of HBO in 66 patients, 51 of whom had severe brain injuries [25]. The HBO treatments were usually given at 2 ATA for 1 hour once or twice daily. However, six treatments were given at 3 ATA for 30 minutes. A total of 143 treatments were given to the 66 patients, but the treatment schedule or number of treatments given to individual patients was not published. During HBO, 33 patients (50%) showed clinical improvement, 21 of them to a remarkable degree. The most impressive effects were increased awareness and responsiveness. Comatose patients rapidly became responsive to painful stimuli and simple commands, but most of these responses were temporary, and regression occurred immediately after decompression. Three patients permanently benefited from HBO; one of these patients received seven HBO treatments in 5 days, which was well above the average number.

Artu et al attempted a prospective controlled study of the effect of HBO in 60 severely brain-injured patients [26]. They were unable to demonstrate any statistically significant differences in the treated versus control group except in patients less than 30 years old who had a brain stem contusion without supertentorial mass lesion. There were several problems with this study. Treatments were administered at 2.5 ATA for 60 minutes, which resulted in the interruption of treatment of 11 patients because of pulmonary difficulties. Additionally, there was an average time delay of 4.5 days before HBO treatment was instituted. This seems to be the critical time for the development of cerebral edema and increased ICP. As previously mentioned, 2.5 ATA does not provide optimal cerebral glucose metabolism or ICP reduction.

Sukoff and Ragatz reported on 50 patients with traumatic cerebral edema who were treated with HBO [12]. Their results with ICP monitoring in 10 patients were discussed previously. In most of these 10 patients, clinical improvement during and following treatment was observed. In the group of 40 HBO patients without ICP monitoring, 22 improved while undergoing their treatments. However, information such as scores on the Glasgow Outcome Scale (GOS) or data from control groups was not given.

A clinical trial conducted in Germany in 1974 strongly suggests that HBO, applied systematically, may improve outcome in severe brain injuries [27]. Of 99 patients with a traumatic midbrain syndrome, every other patient was treated with HBO. The overall mortality for the 49 treated patients was 33%; that for the 50 control patients was 74% (chi-square test: $P \leq 0.01$). Those patients less than 30 years old who had cerebral contusions particularly benefited. Functional outcome also improved: 33% of the HBO-treated patients made a good recovery, whereas only 6% of the control patients did so (one-tailed Fisher's exact: $P \leq 0.01$). Careful analysis of the data reveals that there were more contusions (36%) in the HBO-treated group than in the control group (28%), and the mortality rate for the control patients with contusions (82%) was exceedingly high. This raises questions regarding the randomization process.

In summary, there is clinical and experimental evidence that HBO may be beneficial in the treatment of severe brain injury. Existing studies are not fully convincing; most have been poorly controlled or the treatment assignment was not randomized, and functional recovery and neuropsychological testing were not used to help determine outcome. A review of the literature led us to initiate a controlled, randomized, prospective study to learn whether HBO benefits the severely brain-injured patient.

PROTOCOL

A protocol has been established for the treatment of all severely brain-injured patients: HBO treated, control, or nonrandomized. All patients receive intensive neurosurgical care; the only variable is the HBO delivered to those in the treatment group. Management includes stabilization, CT scanning, neurosurgery as necessary, medical management, and ICP monitoring. Every surviving patient is followed up for at least 18 months to determine functional and neuropsychological recovery.

Subjects

Potential candidates for this study include all victims of severe, closed-head-injury trauma whose Glasgow Coma Score (GCS) is 9 or less (Table 6.1) Patients with positive alcohol or drug levels are reevaluated in 12 hours; those with gunshot wounds are excluded, as are patients with absent brain function persisting for 6 hours. The randomization process is stratified according to age

Table 6.1 Glasgow Coma Score (GCS) at Entry into Study

	No. of Patients		
GCS	*HBO*[a]	*Control*	*Total*
3	3	2	5
4	8	7	15
5	4	5	9
6	6	9	15
7	13	12	25
8	4	3	7
9	6	3	9
Total	44	41	85

[a]HBO = hyperbaric oxygen treatment.

and GCS at time of entry into the study. Patients are not randomized into the study during the 6 hours following hospital admission because rapid neurological improvement or deterioration often occurs at this time. A patient who enters the hospital with a mild or moderate brain injury and subsequently deteriorates to a GCS of 9 or less becomes a candidate for the study, and a signed informed consent is sought.

If a patient meets the neurologic criteria of the study but consent cannot be obtained or there are contraindications to HBO, the patient is followed up as part of the "nonrandomized parallel-protocol" group. Twenty-six patients are in this group; the most common reason has been family refusal to give consent. Nevertheless, the receptiveness of the families to the study has been good.

HBO Treatment

HBO treatments are given in a Sechrist monoplace chamber. Compression to 1.5 ATA occurs at a rate of 1 lb/in^2 per minute and takes 8 minutes to reach depth. Treatments use 100% oxygen, are given every 8 hours, and continue for 2 weeks or until the patient is brain dead or awake and following simple commands.

Complications of HBO Therapy

Complications have pressure-duration (oxygen toxicity) or pressure-volume (barotrauma) relationships. Manifestations of oxygen toxicity in this patient population have involved the respiratory and central nervous systems. Pulmonary oxygen toxicity has most often been characterized by progressively decreased P levels of oxygen tension (Po_2) after repeated exposure to HBO. If a patient requires a fraction of inspired oxygen (Fio_2) of 50% or greater to maintain adequate oxygenation (Po_2 >70 mm Hg) or has progressive changes in chest roentgenograms suggesting oxygen toxicity, HBO therapy is temporarily discontinued. If the patient's condition improves and the Fio_2 requirement becomes 40% or less, treatment is resumed. However if oxygen requirements again increase to an Fio_2 greater than 50%, treatment is permanently terminated. Vitamin E, an antioxidant that may reduce oxygen toxicity, is given every 8 hours [28].

Seizures, a manifestation of oxygen toxicity of the central nervous system, do occur despite routine phenytoin sodium (Dilantin) loading. They are treated acutely with intravenous diazepam (Valium), and HBO is temporarily discontinued until additional phenytoin sodium can be infused. If recurrent seizures develop in patients with HBO despite maximal medical treatment, the HBO therapy is discontinued. If a patient's GCS *motor* score deteriorates by 1 without an explanation, HBO is terminated.

Because the volume of a gas decreases during compression and expands during decompression, any gas-filled cavities in the body are affected and barotrauma may result. In our experience, the most common pressure-volume problems have related to the middle ear. Because these comatose patients are unable to equalize pressure changes in the middle ear, bilateral myringotomies are routinely performed to preclude traumatic rupture of the tympanic membranes.

Initially, each patient is intubated and placed on a ventilator. While in the hyperbaric chamber, a Sechrist time-cycled, flow-generated ventilator is used: tidal volume is determined by flow-time ratio. The cuffs of the endotracheal or tracheostomy tubes are inflated with normal saline before HBO to accommodate for the gas-volume changes. After HBO treatment, the saline is removed and the cuffs are reinflated with air.

Safety

Patient monitoring and safety within the HBO chamber is of the utmost importance. Arterial blood pressure, electrocardiogram, and ICP are routinely monitored, and Swan-Ganz pressure and electroencephalogram have occasionally been monitored during HBO treatments. The ICP is recorded every 10 minutes while the patient is in the chamber.

An intensive care nurse trained in HBO administration is with the patient constantly. Neurosurgical staff, HBO engineers, and respiratory therapists are readily available. Although physical access to the patient is limited during HBO treatment, the chamber can be vented, in an emergency, in approximately 5 seconds. Because fire is a potential hazard, a specially designed room adjacent to the intensive care unit has been constructed to meet strict fire codes. It has its own alarm and water-deluge system. The Sechrist monoplace chamber has an exceedingly safe fire record.

Assessment

At 6, 12, and 18 months after brain injury, survivors are assessed in a "blinded" fashion by a neurologist or, in the case of pediatric patients, a pediatric neurologist. Each patient receives a 100-point neurological examination and is assigned a GOS score. Good recovery or moderate disability is denoted by "favorable recovery" (ability to live independently); severe disability, vegetative state, or death is indicated by "unfavorable recovery." Neuropsychological evaluations are performed at 3 and 12 months postinjury.

CT

Six months after injury, a noncontrast CT scan of the head is done to evaluate the degree of atrophy or encephalomalacia and to exclude communicating hydrocephalus.

Multimodal Evoked Potentials

Brain stem auditory evoked potentials (BAEPs) and short latency somatosensory evoked potentials (SSEPs) are obtained within the first few days after injury and again in 2 weeks. Standard recording procedures are used [29]. Results are graded prospectively. For BAEPs, grade I indicates normal morphology and interpeak latencies; grade II indicates prolonged brain stem transmission but normal morphology; grade III refers to abnormalities in both morphology and central transmission latency; and in grade IV results, only wave 1, corresponding to the auditory nerve itself, is recordable. For SSEPs, grade I indicates normal results; grade II is used when hemispheral potentials are present but delayed referable to the spinal cord potentials; grade III refers to results in which one of the hemispheral potentials is absent; and in grade IV results, both hemispheral potentials are absent.

Neuropsychology

Each patient entering the study is monitored regularly by the neuropsychology service to determine the appropriateness of formal testing. A patient who is fully conscious, verbal, and willing to answer simple questions is screened with the Galveston Orientation and Amnesia Test (a brief survey of orientation and memory for events surrounding the injury) [30]. Patients who score above the impaired range (a score of 66 or greater) are scheduled for neuropsychological testing at 3 and 12 months postinjury. Before testing, premorbid full-scale intelligence quotient (IQ) scores are estimated using the formula derived by Wilson et al based on patient age, sex, occupation, and level of education [31]. Assuming the patient is fully cooperative, the entire neuropsychological test battery is administered at each test date. Current neuropsychological test data are examined in terms of absolute performance levels and estimated premorbid IQs. The result of the IQ testing at month 12 were compared with premorbid intelligence estimates as a general measure of recovery. The test battery was designed to minimize verbal responding while still assessing both language-mediated and nonverbal intellectual skills. The entire battery takes 90 minutes or less to complete for most patients at 3 months post-injury. The testing session at month 12 is longer because a complete Wechsler Adult Intelligence Scale is added to the test battery. The following tests are included: pointing digit span, visual form discriminations [32], full range picture vocabulary test

[33], asphasia screening test [34], Kohs block design test, verbal fluency [35], simple reaction time, trial-making test [36], Rey auditory-verbal learning test [37], Wechsler Adult Intelligence Scale, and the neurobehavior rating scale [38].

STUDY ANALYSIS

The subjects are divided into broad age categories: 0 to 29 years, 30 to 59 years, and 60 years or older. Unlike completely random assignment, this method provides a degree of protection against the chance development of serious age differences between treatment and control groups; such differences could confound a treatment effect.

The GCS strata include individual initial scores of 3 through 6 and those 7 through 9. This gives some protection against the chance development of significant unbalance in initial severity of injury between treatment and control groups.

To maintain a clear randomization process, other notable variables, such as mass lesion versus diffuse lesion, cause of injury, and gender were not included as stratification variables but will be considered as breakdown variables or covariants in the data analysis.

Although the subjects are examined at several times during their recovery, comparisons will be based on the 1-year followup. Separate tests are conducted for the treatment effect in subjects with initial values of 3 through 6 and of 7 through 9. The stratum of subjects with an initial GCS of 4 through 6 is expected to be the more numerous and the more sensitive to the potential benefits of HBO treatment. For this stratum, an increase by 30% in the proportion of favorable recovery will be detected (with a one-tailed alpha of 0.05) 80% of the time with 40 HBO subjects and 40 controls. This is the key comparison of the study. The chi-square statistic will be computed from a contingency table constructed from these data.

PRELIMINARY RESULTS

Eighty-five patients have entered the study during the first 38 months: 44 in the HBO treatment group and 41 in the control group. Three patients in the treatment group did not receive HBO because contraindications were not recognized before the randomization process: one had an unstable cervical fracture, another had an unstable femoral fracture with injury to the femoral artery, and the third had major subcutaneous emphysema. For outcome analysis these patients are considered to have received HBO treatment. Data from the nonrandomized parallel group were not used in this analysis.

Only minor differences exist between the treatment and control groups in terms of gender and cause of injury. In the entire group of 85 patients, 30 suffered multiple injuries (35%). The incidence of multiple injuries in the HBO-treated group was 30%; in the control group it was 41%. Surgical mass lesions occurred in 42% of the 85 patients, with a 36% incidence in the HBO group and a 49% incidence in the control group. The frequency and amounts of mannitol and pentobarbital given in the two groups were similar.

Forty-one patients have received 819 individual HBO treatments: an average of 20 per patient. Among the 41 patients, 8 persistently required an FIO_2 greater than 50%. HBO treatments were temporarily discontinued and then resumed in six of these patients. In two patients there were changes in chest roentgenograms associated with the elevated FIO_2 requirements, and HBO was permanently discontinued. In two patients generalized seizures developed during the HBO treatment despite phenytoin sodium loading. The seizures were treated with intravenous diazepam, the current HBO treatments were halted, additional phenytoin sodium was administered, and HBO treatments were later resumed in both patients. In one patient a hemotympanum developed during an HBO treatment. There has been no apparent neurological deterioration in the first 41 patients treated with HBO attributable to the HBO treatment.

The mortality rate for the 84 patients (1 patient had not been discharged at the time of this analysis) at hospital discharge was 21% (Table 6.2). This had increased to 32% of the 75 patients followed up for 6 months. Favorable recovery occurred in only 26% of 84 patients at the time of discharge, but 51% had obtained this status by 6 months (Table 6.2). Of the 49 patients alive at 12 months, there was only 1 in a persistent vegetative state.

At least one evoked potential battery (including both BAEP and SSEP studies) was obtained on 78 of the 85 patients. Fifty-one patients were given more than one battery of studies. Using the initial study for each patient, prognostic strength of evoked potentials was found to be limited. For BAEP, abnormalities in both morphology and brain stem transmission time (grade III) or absence of potentials after wave 1 (grade IV) presaged an unfavorable

Table 6.2   Outcome in Patients Studied

| | No. of Patients[b] | | |
Time[a]	*Favorable Recovery*	*Deaths*	*Total*
0	22 (26)	18 (21)	84
1	22 (26)	19 (23)	84
3	36 (46)	24 (31)	78
6	38 (51)	24 (32)	75
12	35 (51)	24 (35)	69

[a]Months after discharge from hospital.
[b]Values in parentheses represent percentage of total.

outcome. Only six such studies were encountered (1 HBO-treated patient, 5 control patients), and 5 of the 6 patients had an unfavorable outcome. For SSEPs, bilateral absence of hemispheral potentials (grade IV) seemed to be strongly predictive of an unfavorable outcome. Ten of the 12 patients (9 HBO-treated and 3 control patients) with this initial SSEPs pattern had an unfavorable outcome. Evoked potentials that were less severely abnormal were not necessarily predictive of a favorable or unfavorable outcome.

To date, complete neuropsychologic testing has been conducted on 17 patients. This relatively low number reflects the fact that many of the more severely injured patients are not recovered to a level appropriate for formal neuropsychologic testing by 3 months postinjury. An additional 5 patients have been tested at month 12 but cannot be included in any formal analysis due to the absence of baseline testing. Of the 17 patients for whom complete data are available, 8 were in the GCS range from 4 through 6 at the time of entry into the study. Of these 8, 7 were in the "favorable recovery" group at month 12. The eighth patient was treated with HBO and was severely disabled at 12 months postinjury. Results available to date are not sufficient to allow a systematic comparison of neuropsychologic outcome in patients treated with HBO versus control.

When the entry GCS and the 6-month outcome are analyzed, a clear correlation is anticipated ($P = 0.04$). Recovery at 6 months was also analyzed comparing two age groups: patients less than 30 years old had a statistically significant improved outcome compared with patients greater than 30 years ($P = 0.004$). Again as anticipated, patients harboring mass lesions requiring surgical treatment fared significantly worse than patients with diffuse, non-surgical lesions ($P = 0.004$). Analyses of our data indicate that our overall mortality and recovery rates compare favorably with those of other medical centers (Table 6.3).

ICPs were monitored in 82 of the 85 patients. Sixty patients had bilateral ICP monitoring as part of a study to evaluate the relative accuracy of ventriculostomies, subdural catheters, and subarachnoid bolts [39]. An analysis of the ICP data in the 41 patients treated in the hyperbaric chamber reveals a trend toward increased ICP during the acute treatment, with a tendency to revert to pretreatment baseline values within an hour or two of ending the HBO treatment (Figure 6.1).

There are several apparent causes of the relative increase in ICP during HBO treatment. The first is that, although the patients' heads are routinely elevated 30 degrees while in the intensive care unit, this must be reduced to about 10 degrees during the HBO treatment. Second, even though the compression time of 1 lb/in² per minute is relatively slow, agitation and restlessness in many patients appears to contribute to ICP elevations. This agitation may be due to middle ear discomfort (see "Complications" above). Myringotomies, sedation, and muscle relaxants seem to have helped this problem. Another possible cause of elevated ICPs was the problem of equalizing the pressures in

Table 6.3   Review of Severe Brain Trauma Series

Medical Center [Reference]	Patients			Outcome			
	n	OR (%)[a]	Multiple Trauma (%)	Time After Discharge (mo)	Favorable (%)[b]	Unfavorable (%)[c]	Mortality (%)
Hennepin County	85	42	35	6	51	49	32
Glasgow [40]	593	54	32	6	41	59	48
Richmond [41]	158	44	48	3	47	53	40
Penn [42]	1107	44	—	3	42	58	41

[a]Patients harboring mass lesions requiring surgical treatment.
[b]Good recovery or moderate disability.
[c]Severe disability, vegetative state, or death.

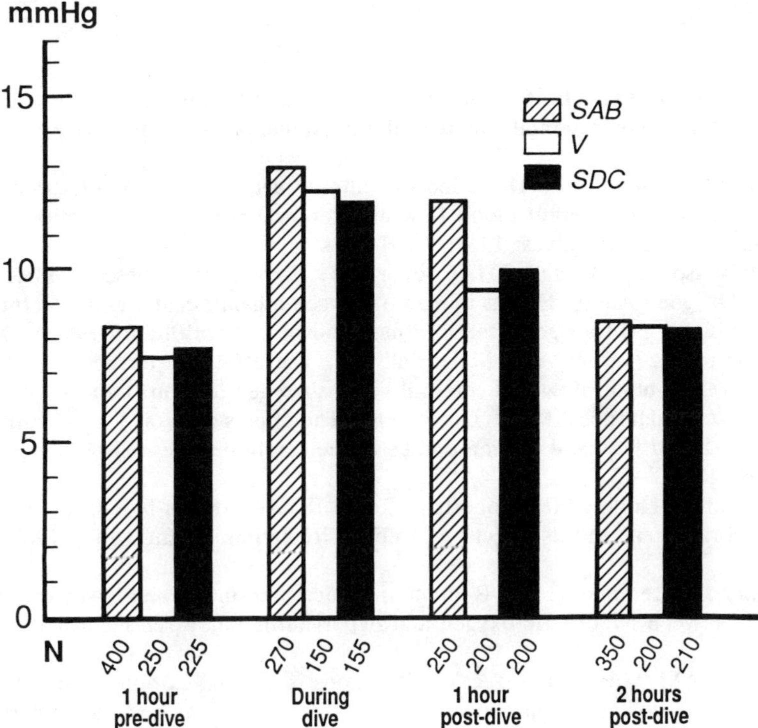

Figure 6.1   Mean intracranial pressure values of patients treated with hyperbaric oxygen. Monitoring was done with subarachnoid bolts (SAB), ventriculotomies (V), and subdural catheters (SDC).

the pressure transducers at the same rate that the hyperbaric chamber was pressurized. Because of the relatively rapid changes in atmospheric pressure during treatment, any obstruction encountered in the transducer ventilatory tube resulted in inaccurate ICPs. This problem has been resolved by shortening the ventilatory tubes. In addition, proper placement of the transducer in relation to the ICP monitor remains critical for accuracy.

Analysis of the 85 patients entered into the study has shown that HBO can safely and systematically be applied to severely brain-injured patients. Moreover, outcome analysis of the 85 patients reveals a satisfactory overall mortality as well as recovery. This outcome is periodically analyzed by observers not directly involved with the study in terms of HBO versus the control group. There has been no suggestion of a harmful effect from the HBO. It is anticipated that at least another 85 patients must be studied to render a statistically significant conclusion regarding the efficacy of treating severely brain-injured patients with HBO.

REFERENCES

1. Miller JD. The effects of hyperbaric oxygen at 2 and 3 atmospheres and intravenous mannitol on experimentally increased intracranial pressure. Eur Neurol 1973;10:1–11.
2. Kety SS, Schmidt CF. The effects of altered arterial tensions of carbon dioxide and oxygen on cerebral blood flow and cerebral oxygen consumption of normal young men. J Clin Invest 1948;27:484–92.
3. Lambertson CJ, Kough RH, Cooper DY, Emmel BL, Loeschke HH, Schmidt CF. Oxygen toxicity: Effects in man of oxygen inhalation at 1 and 3.5 atmospheres upon blood gas transport, cerebral metabolism. J Appl Physiol 1953;5:471–86.
4. Jacobson K, Harper AM, McDowall DG. The effects of oxygen under pressure on cerebral blood-flow and cerebral venous oxygen tension. Lancet 1963;2:549.
5. Jacobson I, Harper AM, McDowall DG. The effects of O_2 at 1 and 2 atmospheres on the blood flow and oxygen uptake of the cerebral cortex. Surg Gynecol Obstet 1964;119:737–42.
6. Reivich M, Holling HE, Roberts B, Toale JF. Reversal of blood flow through the vertebral artery and its effect on cerebral circulation. N Eng J Med 1961;265:878–85.
7. Miller JD, Ledingham IM. Reduction of increased intracranial pressure. Comparison between hyperbaric oxygen and hyperventilation. Arch Neurol 1971;24:210–16.
8. Harper AM, Glass HI. Effect of alterations in arterial carbon dioxide tension on the blood flow through the cerebral cortex at normal and low arterial blood pressures. J Neurol Neurosurg Psychiatry 1965;28:449–52.
9. Miller JD, Fitch W, Ledingham IM, Jennett WB. The effect of hyperbaric oxygen on experimentally increased intracranial pressure. J Neurosurg 1970;33:287–96.
10. Kanai N, Hayakawa T, Mogami H. Blood flow changes in carotid and vertebral arteries by hyperbaric oxygenation. Neurology (Minneapolis) 1973;23:159–63.
11. Nagao S, Okumura S, Nishimoto A. Effects of hyperbaric oxygenation on cerebral vasomotor tone in acute intracranial hypertension: an experimental study. Resuscitation 1975;4:51–59.
12. Sukoff MH, Ragatz RE. Hyperbaric oxygenation for the treatment of acute cerebral edema. Neurosurgery 1982;10:29–38.
13. Hayakawa T, Kanai N, Kuroda R, Yamada R, Mogami H. Response of cerebrospinal fluid pressure to hyperbaric oxygenation. J Neurol Neurosurg Psychiatry 1971;34:580–86.
14. Holbach KH, Caroli A, Wassmann H. Cerebral energy metabolism in patients with brain lesions at normo- and hyperbaric oxygen pressures. J Neurol 1977;217:17–30.
15. Artu F, Philippon B, Gau F, Berger M, Deleuze R. Cerebral blood flow, cerebral metabolism and cerebrospinal fluid biochemistry in brain-injured patients after exposure to hyperbaric oxygen. Eur Neurol 1976;14:351–64.
16. Langfitt TW, Kassell NF. Acute brain swelling in neurosurgical patients. J Neurosurg 1966;24:975–83.
17. Langfitt TW, Weinstein JD, Kassell NF. Cerebral vasomotor paralysis produced by intracranial hypertension. Neurology (Minneapolis) 1965;15:622–41.

18. Grahm DI, Adams JH. Ischemic brain damage in fatal head injuries. Lancet 1971;1:265–66.
19. Lewin W. Vascular lesions in head injuries. Brit J Surg 1968;55:321–31.
20. Bruce DA, Langfitt TW, Miller JD, Schutz H, Vapulahti MP, Stanek A, Goldberg HI. Regional cerebral blood flow, intracranial pressure and brain metabolism in comatose patients. J Neurosurg 1973;38:131–44.
21. Sukoff MH, Hollin SA, Espinosa OE, Jacobson JH. The protective effect of hyperbaric oxygenation in experimental cerebral edema. J Neurosurg 1968;29:236–41.
22. Sperl MP Jr, Svien HJ, Goldstein NP, Kernohan JW, Grindlay JH. Experimental production of local cerebral edema by an expanding intracerebral mass. Proc Staff Meet Mayo Clin 1957;32:744–49.
23. Sukoff MH, Hollin SA, Jacobson JH. The protective effect of hyperbaric oxygenation in experimentally produced cerebral edema and compression. Surgery 1967;62:40–46.
24. Moody RA, Mead CO, Ruamsuke S, Mullan S. Therapeutic value of oxygen at normal and hyperbaric pressure in experimental head injury. J Neurosurg 1970;32:51–54.
25. Mogami H, Hayakawa T, Kanai N, Kuroda R, Yamada R, Ikeda T, Katsurada K, Sugimoto T. Clinical application of hyperbaric oxygenation in the treatment of acute cerebral damage. J Neurosurg 1969;31:636–43.
26. Artu F, Charcornac R, Deleuze R. Hyperbaric oxygenation for severe head injuries. Preliminary results of a controlled study. Eur Neurol 1976;14:310–18.
27. Holback KH, Wassman H, Kolberg T. Verbesserte reversibilitat des traumatischen mittelhumsyndroms bei anwendung des hyperbaren oxygemerung. Acta neurochi 1974;30:247–56.
28. Sanders, AP, Gelein RS, Currie WD. The effect of hyperbaric oxygenation on the metabolism of the lung. In: Lambertsen CJ, ed. Underwater physiology. V. Proceedings of the fifth symposium on underwater physiology. Bethesda, MD: FASEB, 1976;483–92.
29. Anderson DC, Bundlie S, Rockswold GL. Multimodality evoked potentials in closed head trauma. Arch Neurol 1984;41:369–74.
30. Levin HS, O'Donnel VM, Grossman RG. The Galveston Orientation and Amnesia Test. A practical scale to assess cognition after head injury. J Nerv Ment Dis 1979;167:675–84.
31. Wilson RS, Rosenbaum G, Brown G, Rourke D, Whitman D, Grisell J. An index of premorbid intelligence. J Consult Clin Psychol 1978;46:1554–55.
32. Benton AL, Hamsher K deS, Barney NR, Spreen O. Contributions to neuropsychological assessment: A clinical manual. New York: Oxford University Press, 1983.
33. Ammons RB, Ammons CH. Use and evaluation of full-range picture vocabulary test: Partial summary through March 1976: Vol I. Published papers. Percept Mot Skills 1977;45:999–1002.
34. Halstead WC, Wepman JM. The Halstead-Wepman aphasia screening test. J Spch Hear Disord 1959;14:9–15.
35. Spreen O, Benton A. Neurosensory center comprehensive examination for aphasia. University of Victoria, B.C.: Neuropsychological Laboratory Department of Psychology, 1969.

36. Reitan RM. Validity of the Trail Making Test as an indication of organic brain damage. Percept Mot Skills 1958;8:271–76.
37. Rey. L'examen clinique en psychologie. Paris: Presses Universitaires de France, 1964.
38. Levin HS, Overall JE, Goethe KE, High W, Sisson RA. Neurobehavioral Rating Scale. Galveston, TX; 1983. Unpublished.
39. Mollman HD, Rockswold GL, Ford SE: A clinical comparison of subarachnoid catheters to ventriculostomies and subarachnoid bolts. A prospective study. J Neurosurg 1988;68(5):737–41.
40. Jennet B, Teasdale G, Braakman R, Heiden J, Kurze T. Prognosis of patients with severe head injury. Neurosurgery 1979;4:283–89.
41. Miller JD, Butterworth JF, Gudeman SK, Faulkner JE, Choi SC, Selhorst JB, Harbison JW, Lutz HA, Young HF, Becker DP. Further experience in the management of severe head injury. J Neurosurg 1981;54:289–99.
42. Gennaralli TA, Spielman GM, Langfi HTW, Gildenberg PL, Harrington T, Jane JA, Marshall CF, Miller JE, Pitts LH. Influence of the type of intracranial lesion on outcome from severe head injury. A multicenter approach using a new classification system. J Neurosurg 1982;56:26–32.

Chapter 7

Controversies in the Use of Anticonvulsants to Prevent Posttraumatic Epilepsy

L. James Willmore

One aspect of the management of severe head trauma requires a decision about whether to treat a patient with anticonvulsant medication. If the patient is to be given a prophylactic anticonvulsant, then an appropriate drug must be selected. The treating physician intends to prevent the occurrence of a convulsive seizure after injury or after an operative procedure. Although no specific clinical studies are available, it is intuitive that the occurrence of convulsive seizures, with associated hypoxemia, altered blood pressure, and altered brain metabolism, would complicate or aggravate secondary effects of severe head trauma. It has been estimated that at least 60% of patients with serious brain injury will be given an anticonvulsant drug some time during evaluation or treatment [1].

To *prevent* means to keep from happening, or to render impossible by advanced provisions. The administration of a drug to a head trauma patient with intent to interfere with a process that might intensify the secondary effects of the injury is an example of prevention. If the administration of anticonvulsant drugs is used within the context of prevention of epilepsy, then this implies that epileptogenesis has occurred, and that the medication given is intended to keep the inevitable—a seizure—from happening. This direct rationale can be based upon the predictive information that a given patient with a high risk of having seizures [2] should be treated. The rationalization becomes the following: If there is a direct relationship between head trauma dose and epileptogenesis, then those patients with the most severe injury have the highest risk of having a seizure and should be treated with an anticonvulsant.

In the context cited, prevention is a worthy goal. However, in recent years physicians have administered anticonvulsant drugs to patients with head trauma with the intent of prophylaxis [1,3]. *Prophylaxis* is the art of guarding against or preventing disease, hence prevention of the process of epileptogenesis that might lead to the occurrence of seizures. Because prevention intends to keep a seizure from happening, prophylactic use of an anticonvulsant drug must be thought to interfere with the process of posttraumatic epileptogenesis.

This type of patient management implies the following: that there is knowledge of the process of epileptogenesis induced by trauma; that anticonvulsant drugs will intervene in the process and in the progression of events initiated by brain injury, and that, somehow, the injured brain will not develop clinically manifest epileptiform discharge because of the prophylactic administration of anticonvulsant drug. This is a logical approach, but it may not be correct.

TRAUMA DOSE AND PREDICTIVE FACTORS

The severity of brain injury, reflecting trauma dose, appears to correlate with the incidence of posttraumatic epilepsy (PTE). To classify epilepsy risk, Caveness [4] used six categories of head trauma based upon the severity of injury. Patients in categories I through III had intact dura mater but a spectrum of injury including neurological sequelae and obvious damage to the brain; the incidence of epilepsy in these patients ranged from 7 to 39%, respectively. If the dura was penetrated, producing neurological deficits in some cases, then the incidence of epilepsy ranged from 20 to 57%.

The time of occurrence of the first seizure, although variable, documents a latency that may be related to the injury responses that are critical to the process of epileptogenesis. Of patients in whom PTE develops, 57% will have had their first seizure within 1 year [5]. The timing of the seizure may also be divided into early epilepsy (within the first week) and late epilepsy (beyond the first week) [6]. Management is complicated by immediate seizures, occurring in the first hour after trauma in 30% of such patients [6], and by posttraumatic status epilepticus. In such cases, anticonvulsant medications are administered and an episode of hypoxia may be added to the substrate of problems caused by impact injury. An immediate seizure may occasionally be a signal event denoting the presence of an intracranial hematoma, but has little prognostic effect for late seizures [6,7]. However, the occurrence of a seizure within the first week after injury (an early seizure) has prognostic significance for subsequent seizures. Jennett and Lewin [8] found a fourfold increase in the incidence of late epilepsy in those patients who had an early seizure. Other predictive indicators associated with increased risk of late epilepsy include duration of posttraumatic amnesia beyond 24 hours, the presence of a depressed skull fracture, or the development of an intracranial hematoma [9]. Indeed, mathematical prediction using weighted risk factors allows calculation of liability at the time of injury for development of PTE, or estimation of continued risk at various times after injury [2,10].

PROPHYLAXIS AND PREVENTION

Investigators attempting to answer questions regarding the efficacy of pharmacologic prophylaxis of PTE are confronted by a series of difficult problems in experimental design. A satisfactory answer requires that large numbers of patients be entered in a prospective study with double-blind administration of anticonvulsant or placebo. The investigator must be able to convince patients to comply with medication schedules for many months, and must be able to document compliance by measuring anticonvulsant blood levels. Furthermore, the study must be of sufficient duration to assure that latency to seizure onset following head trauma is embraced by the protocol. Few studies meet these criteria.

Clinical experiments designed to answer the question regarding the efficacy of prophylaxis for PTE fall into three broad categories. The design of reported studies are open, retrospective, or prospective. Variations in these categories include blinded, placebo-controlled, uncontrolled, and historical controls.

Open Studies

The first reports, cited by Rapport and Penry [3] were performed by Hoff and Hoff, by Birkmayer, and by Popek and Musil (Table 7.1). In these studies, phenytoin was used alone, or in combination with phenobarbital. Control

Table 7.1 Efficacy of Prophylaxis for Posttraumatic Epilepsy

		% of Patients Developing Epilepsy	
Studies	*Drug*	*Control*	*Treated*
Open			
Hoff and Hoff[a]	Phenytoin	38	4
Birkmayer[a]	Phenytoin	51	6
Popek and Musil[a]	Phenytoin and phenobarbital	21	0
Young et al [11]	Phenytoin		6
Servit and Musil [12]	Phenytoin and phenobarbital	25	2.1
Retrospective			
Rish and Caveness [13]	Phenytoin	3.7	1.6
Wohns and Wyler [14]	Phenytoin	50	10
Double blind, controlled			
Penry et al [15]	Phenytoin and phenobarbital	13	23
Young et al [16]	Phenytoin	10.8	12.9

[a]Studies mentioned in a review by Rapport and Penry [3].

patients were not given anticonvulsant medication. The studies were open, in that the patient and the investigator knew who was receiving anticonvulsant drugs. The studies reported several years of experience; and it is assumed that anticonvulsant blood levels were not measured. All three studies concluded that prophylactic anticonvulsant administration prevented the development of PTE. Young et al [11] also performed an open, prospective, uncontrolled study. In 6% of their patients who were treated with phenytoin, PTE developed. These investigators documented a significant problem with compliance, particularly after one month of treatment. Comparing their results with a controlled percentage incidence they had constructed from reports in the literature, these investigators concluded that early administration of anticonvulsant drugs prevented the development of PTE. They recommended that patients within a risk category of 15% or more be given phenytoin as a prophylactic measure against PTE. Servit and Musil [12] reported the results of long-term follow-up of head trauma patients treated with a combination of phenytoin and phenobarbital. Follow-up was available between 3 and 10 years after injury. The treated and control groups were not numerically equal. The investigators reported a 25% incidence of PTE in the control group, and a 2.1% incidence in the treated group. Seizures occurring in the treated group occurred only after anticonvulsant therapy had been discontinued for a period of time. Although anticonvulsant blood levels were not measured, this report suggested that a low dose of phenytoin and phenobarbital (a dose not known, when calculated on an anticipated milligram-per-kilogram basis, to produce a therapeutic blood level) is effective in preventing PTE.

Open studies are highly supportive of the hypothesis that the process of epileptogenesis can be interrupted by the administration of anticonvulsant medication.

Retrospective Studies

Rish and Caveness [13] assessed the incidence of early seizures following head trauma in their registry of patients injured in Vietnam. The authors define an early seizure as occurring during the seven days following injury. Although a delay of several days was expected before a steady-state level of anticonvulsant was reached in the blood, these authors could not detect any difference in incidence of early seizures between phenytoin-treated patients and untreated patients after head trauma.

Wohns and Wyler [14] reviewed the records of 62 patients who were at high risk for development of PTE. These patients had one or more critical indicators of a significant trauma dose, including depressed skull fracture, dural or cortical laceration, or an extended period of posttraumatic amnesia. Phenytoin had been given to 50 patients and withheld from 12. PTE developed in five patients in the phenytoin treatment group (10%) and six in the control group (50%). Although it purports to support the hypothesis that administration of anticonvulsant medication will prevent the development of PTE, there are several problems with this study. The authors acknowledge the unequal numbers of treated and untreated patients, and the possible bias in the retrospective selection of the patients at risk. However, of concern is the fact that the number of patients not included in the study exceeds the number included by a factor of 4.

Double-Blind Studies

One early effort to obtain objective information regarding the question of prophylaxis of PTE was published in abstract form by Perry et al [15]. This 36-month study involved administration of phenytoin and phenobarbital. A control group was used. Although specific information was limited by the use of the abstract format, the investigators observed a 21% and 13% probability of seizure in the treated and control groups, respectively. The authors report that no significant difference was calculated between the treatment and the control groups. This study appears to suggest that administration of anticonvulsant medication had no effect on the incidence of PTE in the treatment group.

Young et al [16] followed 179 brain-injured patients for 18 months. They administered phenytoin in a prospective, double-blind, placebo-controlled fashion. Patients were given loading and maintenance doses of phenytoin and were followed with measurement of anticonvulsant blood levels. The treated group consisted of 85 patients, and there were 74 placebo-control patients. At the termination of the study, seizures had occurred in 12.9% of the treated patients and in 10.8% of the control patients. The authors suggested that a study of patients with a phenytoin blood level of greater than 12 µg/ml was needed before it could be concluded that prophylactic phenytoin is ineffective in preventing the development of PTE.

WHEN TO DISCONTINUE
ANTICONVULSANT DRUGS

Decisions regarding discontinuation of anticonvulsant drugs in head trauma patients who have been seizure-free appear to be made arbitrarily. Servit and Musil [12] followed a cohort of 143 patients who had been treated at the time of injury with low-dose phenytoin and phenobarbital. They performed electroencephalograms (EEGs) at 3, 6, 12, and 24 months after injury. If, at the end of two years, the EEG failed to reveal an abnormality and the patient had not had amnesia, then medications were tapered over six months. The authors note that 16.2% of patients had EEG abnormalities and thus were presumed to be on continued treatment. Although Young et al [11] did not directly address the issue of when to discontinue anticonvulsants, they reported that few patients continued to take anticonvulsants beyond one month after initial treatment.

No reports exist, but it appears that physicians chose arbitrary times for discontinuation of medication. The choices appear to be 6 months from the time of injury if seizure free, 1 year, or 2 years. EEGs are occasionally used in making the decision, with presumed epileptiform activity being an indication to continue treatment.

SUMMARY

The greatest impediment to prevention of the process of epileptogenesis is lack of knowledge of the mechanism that results in the development or activation of a seizure focus. The common clinical situation of a patient with a trauma dose sufficient to initiate epileptogenesis, and with injury responses that would be worsened by the effects of a convulsive seizure, require practical intervention to protect the patient in this acute setting. If phenytoin or another anticonvulsant is to be administered to prevent a seizure in the time following a severe head injury, then that medication should be administered intravenously, and pharmacologic principles should be obeyed. Such a patient should receive twice the calculated maintenance dose for phenytoin, given intravenously at a rate no greater than 40 mg per minute. The maintenance dose is given intravenously once a day with the knowledge that steady state will be achieved three days after initiation of treatment.

There are no guidelines to determine when the anticonvulsant should be discontinued. If an injured patient has not had a seizure in the early period and continues to be seizure free while on anticonvulsant drugs, then best judgment, without supporting data, would suggest the following plan: (1) Obtain a baseline EEG at one year after injury. (2) Obtain an additional EEG at two years after injury. (3) If the EEG remains free of any sign of epileptiform discharge, then begin tapering of the anticonvulsant drug. (4) If the patient has been operating a motor vehicle, then that patient must stop driving during the subsequent year. (5) Lower phenytoin dose by no more than 25 mg of the total daily dose per month.

Although these recommendations may seem unduly conservative, no information is available to direct the treating physician in this matter. Although the literature suggests that prophylactic use of anticonvulsant drugs will not prevent epileptogenesis, one question remains. If a therapeutic level of 12.5 μg/ml or greater is maintained, there may be an effect on the occurrence of a seizure. If phenytoin is used to prevent seizures, then scrupulous attention is required to maintain therapeutic blood levels and encourage patient compliance. At this time prophylactic administration of an anticonvulsant drug could be reserved for the most seriously injured patients in the time immediately following trauma. No evidence is available to suggest that administration of anticonvulsant drugs to all brain-injured patients will have an impact on the overall incidence of PTE.

REFERENCES

1. Rapport RL, Penry JK. A survey of attitudes toward the pharmacological prophylaxis of posttraumatic epilepsy. J Neurosurg 1973;38:159–66.
2. Feeney DM, Walker AE. The prediction of posttraumatic epilepsy. Arch Neurol 1979;36:8–12.
3. Rapport RL, Penry JK. Pharmacologic prophylaxis of posttraumatic epilepsy: A review. Epilepsia 1972;13:295–304.
4. Caveness WF. Epilepsy, a product of trauma in our time. Epilepsia 1976;17:207–15.
5. Salazar AM, Jabbari B, Vance SC, Grafman J, Amin D, Dillon JD. Epilepsy after penetrating head injury. I. Clinical correlates: A report of the Vietnam Head Injury Study. Neurology 1985;35:1406–14.
6. Jennett B. Early traumatic epilepsy. Incidence and significance after nonmissile injuries. Arch Neurol 1974;30:394–98.
7. Jennett B. Epilepsy and acute traumatic intracranial haematoma. J Neurol Neurosurg Psychiatry 1975;38:378–81.
8. Jennett WB, Lewin W. Traumatic epilepsy after closed head injuries. J Neurol Neurosurg Psychiatry 1960;23:295–301.
9. Jennett B. Epilepsy after nonmissile head injuries. Scot Med J 1973;18:8–13.
10. Weiss GH, Salazar AM, Vance SC, Grafman JH, Jabbari B. Predicting posttraumatic epilepsy in penetrating head injury. Arch Neurol 1986;43:771–73.
11. Young B, Rapp R, Brooks WH, Madauss W, Norton JA. Posttraumatic epilepsy prophylaxis. Epilepsia 1979;20:671–81.
12. Servit Z, Musil F. Prophylactic treatment of posttraumatic epilepsy: Results of a long-term follow-up in Czechoslovakia. Epilepsia 1981;22:315–20.
13. Rish BL, Caveness WF. Relation of prophylactic medication to the occurrence of early seizures following craniocerebral trauma. J Neurosurg 1973;38:155–58.
14. Wohns RNW, Wyler AR. Prophylactic phenytoin in severe head injuries. J Neurosurg 1979;51:507–9.
15. Penry JK, White BG, Brackett CE. A controlled prospective study of the pharmacologic prophylaxis of posttraumatic epilepsy. Neurology 1979;29:600–1.
16. Young B, Rapp RP, Norton JA, Haack KD, Tibbs PA, Bean JR. Failure of prophylactically administered phenytoin to prevent late posttraumatic seizures. J Neurosurg 1983;58:236–41.

Chapter 8

Assessment of Everyday Memory Functioning Following Severe Brain Injury

Barbara Wilson
Janet Cockburn
Alan Baddeley

In the first few days or weeks following a brain injury, relatives are typically concerned with the brain-injured person's survival. When survival is assured, their concern shifts to the physical welfare of their brain-injured relative. Usually, several months pass before relatives show a primary concern for the brain-injured person's cognitive or behavioral impairments. Paradoxically, these are the very impairments that are likely to be the most enduring and the most handicapping for daily living. Of the cognitive problems, memory impairment is probably the most prevalent and disabling, and the most resistant to therapy.

A number of studies have identified weaknesses associated with memory failure following severe brain injury. Brooks [1], for example, found that his patients showed impairment on tests of prose recall, paired-associate learning, and backward digit span. All these tasks require the acquisition of new material and the capacity to hold it while manipulating it into the form needed for response. Although tests of memory failure such as these employed by Brooks and many other investigators are frequently sensitive in detecting organic memory impairment and identifying information processing problems, they are of limited value in informing us about the nature or severity of the memory problems brain-injured people are likely to encounter in their daily lives. Traditional tests do not usually mirror the demands made upon a person's memory in real life; neither do they tell us how brain-injured persons might attempt to cope with the problems they are faced with from day to day. Such tests do not enable us to distinguish the patient's (or relative's) own priorities in remembering; these may be characterized by painful, indistinct desires to achieve at least some control over memory that assists the business of daily living. Furthermore, traditional tests may be insensitive to changes in memory functioning over time or after therapy; their psychometric measures are poor at teasing out practice effects of repeated testing, and they can easily miss genuine functional changes or coping skills.

Because memory impairment may be a major constraint on rehabilitation, adequate assessment of everyday memory is potentially important in determining both specific treatment objectives and measurement of change over time. There are many reasons why one would conduct a memory assessment. It might be in the cause of proving or disproving a theoretical point; it might be aimed at determining whether a person's memory functioning is in the abnormal range, or at establishing a comparative score with peers; and it might be aimed at finding out whether a person has difficulties with global or material specific memory.

Important as these purposes are, they are not high among the priorities of brain-injured people themselves, their relatives, or rehabilitation staff working to achieve some degree of improvement in the powers of remembering of a particular brain-injured patient. All too often, psychological assessment reports are filed away, elucidating little if anything about the brain-injured person's predicament. It has been frequently observed that a mismatch exists between the information a psychologist provides and the information required by almost everyone else.

A typical psychological report states the scores obtained by a patient in a series of tests, states whether these scores are in the impaired range, sometimes includes the means and standard deviations of the general population, and indicates, when known, how the scores have changed since a previous assessment. The report might receive a glance or two before being filed away. Sometimes patients, relatives, or therapists may challenge the psychologist to relate the assessment findings to everyday life. For example, the occupational therapist might ask, "What does it mean when you state that X's Rey Osterreith recall is impaired?" or "How will Y's chances of returning to work be affected by the fact that he cannot do paired-associate learning?" A relative might say, "I know she cannot do your memory tests, but she remembers things that interest her and she's never going to need to remember lists or funny figures when she gets home."

There has been a failure to apply psychological and neuropsychological understanding and skills to the predicaments faced by the brain-injured population as they attempt to make sense of their daily world. We have for too long ignored the context in which impairments find expression. However, new interest is developing in everyday memory within the academic world, particularly in Britain, and it is reflected in attempts to bring psychology out of the laboratory. For example, Harris and Morris [2] cover a wide range of everyday memory topics, such as remembering our way around a terrain [3], remembering to do things [4], and remembering our classmates at school [5].

Some effort has been made to apply the procedures for measuring everyday memory to the brain-injured population (see Sunderland et al [6], for example). Over the past four years we have been examining a number of procedures to assess everyday memory functioning in a group of brain-injured people attending Rivermead Rehabilitation Centre in Oxford, England.

SELF-REPORT MEASURES

Studies attempting to measure everyday memory problems by using self-report measures, such as rating scales, questionnaires, and checklists, have found poor agreement between these and traditional or laboratory tasks. The latter measure performance on artificial material (examples being lists of unrelated words or abstract designs). Sunderland et al [7] designed a study to evaluate the relationship between laboratory tests of memory and subjective reports of memory difficulties by brain-injured people and their relatives. Questionnaires were used to investigate the type and frequency of memory lapses noticed in everyday life after a severe brain injury. Correlations with objective tests were low. However, relatives' responses were more valid (determined by the relationship to objective laboratory tests) as measures of memory ability than responses by the patients themselves. This, they suggest, is because severely impaired patients cannot recall their own failures. Few subjects, however, were reported to be seriously handicapped by memory failures at the time the questionnaires were completed. A related study [6] found that daily checklists kept by patients related better to objective test results than did responses to questionnaires, possibly because filling in a checklist provides a more immediate evaluation of problems.

Another study that used a rating scale was reported by Kapur and Pearson [8]. The items were derived from reports of memory difficulties received from neurological patients. They subsequently found good agreement between responses of brain-injured patients and their relatives but, again, little correlation with objective tests of memory. Their subjects, too, were reported to be relatively mildly impaired.

Although lack of insight among brain-injured patients into their own problems may be an important factor in the poor agreement between self-report and objective test results, it is also possible that the tests do not reflect the types of memory problems that actually affect everyday behavior.

The first study of ours to be reported here looked at a group of 23 severely brain-injured patients, all of whom had been in coma for at least 48 hours. We wanted to know whether these patients had good insight into their memory problems. We asked the brain-injured patients, and asked their relatives, to rate the memory difficulties experienced by the brain injured; we also asked the therapists involved in treatment to record any memory failures occurring during therapy.

During the second and third weeks following admission to the rehabilitation center, patients were asked to complete a ten-item rating scale based on the one devised by Kapur and Pearson [8]. Patients were asked to indicate for each item whether, in comparison with their pre-accident ability, their memory was "about the same" (score 0), "slightly worse" (score 1), or "very much worse" (score 2). The maximum total score was thus 20. A member of the family of each patient was also asked to complete an identical scale for his or her brain-injured relative. The rating scale is shown in Table 8.1.

In addition, therapists were asked to complete checklists on each patient for two weeks. The checklists were modified from those of Sunderland et al [6,7,9]. Therapists were asked to note examples of forgetting by patients in three main areas: forgetting things, in conversation, and actions. There are 19 subheadings within these areas (Table 8.2). Because patients at Rivermead have about five hours of therapy each day, much detailed information on the type and frequency of everyday memory problems was gathered.

All the patients were brain-injured people admitted to Rivermead during an eight-month period. There were 18 male and 5 female patients, aged 14 to 63 years (mean age, 30.39 years $\pm$ 12.06 standard deviation [SD]). The length of coma ranged from 2 days to 6 months, and time postinjury ranged from 1 month to 7 years (mean, 19 months $\pm$ 22 SD). The group could be described as a typical mixed-gender group found in a British rehabilitation center.

Table 8.1 Memory Rating Scale[a]

	Rating[b]		
Item to Remember	*About the Same*	*Slightly Worse*	*Very Much Worse*
(1) The date	0	1	2
(2) The month	0	1	2
(3) The names of people you have known for a long time	0	1	2
(4) The names of people you have met once or twice	0	1	2
(5) The faces of people you have known for a long time	0	1	2
(6) The faces of people you have met once or twice	0	1	2
(7) How to get somewhere	0	1	2
(8) Where you have put something	0	1	2
(9) What you have been told	0	1	2
(10) What you have read	0	1	2

[a]Based on scale devised by Kapur and Pearson [7].
[b]Memory compared with that before brain injury.

Table 8.2 Memory Checklist[a]

| Patient __________________________ | Department _________________________ |
| Date ______________________________ | Filled in by _______________________ |

| | 9:00 | 10:45 | 1:30 | 3:15 |
| | 10:30 | 12:00 | 3:00 | 4:00 |

A. Forgetting things. Did s/he:

  (1) Forget things s/he *was told* yesterday or a few days ago and have to be reminded of them?

  (2) Forget where s/he had *put something* or lose things around the department?

  (3) Forget *where* things are *normally kept* or look for things in the wrong places?

  (4) Forget *when* something had happened, for instance whether it was yesterday or last week?

  (5) Forget *to take things* with him/her, or leave things behind and have to go back for them?

  (6) Forget *to do things* s/he said s/he would do?

  (7) Forget *important details* of what s/he had done the day before?

  (8) Forget *details* of his/her daily *routine?*

  (9) Forget a *change* in his/her *daily routine?*

 (10) Forget the *names* of people s/he has met before?

B. Conversation. Did s/he:

 (11) *Ramble on* about unimportant or irrelevant events?

 (12) Find words on *the tip of the tongue,* knowing the word but not quite able to produce it?

 (13) Get *details* of what someone has said confused?

 (14) Tell a *story or joke* s/he has told before?

 (15) Forget what s/he had already said, perhaps *repeating what s/he has just said* or saying "What was I talking about?"?

C. Actions. Did s/he:

 (16) Have difficulty with *picking up a new skill,* e.g., playing a game or learning to use a new gadget?

 (17) *Check up* on whether s/he had done things s/he intended to do?

 (18) *Get lost* on a journey or in a building where s/he has been before?

 (19) Forget what s/he was originally doing *after becoming distracted* by something else?

No. of patients seen in session ________________________________

Any other comments or observations ____________________________

[a]Modified from checklist of Sunderland et al [6].

Results

People who thought their memory functioning was very much worse than before their accident would score in the region of 20 points, and those who believed they were just as good as before their accident scored 0. The maximum number of memory failures during the two-week period that could be reported by therapists was 760 (19 items, 4 sessions each day, 10 therapy days). The mean scores of patients, relatives, and therapists are shown in Table 8.3.

The correlations between these measures can be seen in Table 8.4. Time postonset has also been included, because it was thought that this factor might possibly influence subjective rating (as it had in a study by Sunderland et al [6]). Correlations were also calculated with age, but because all were so close to 0 they have been excluded from the table.

The high correlation between the ratings made by the brain-injured patients and the ratings made by their relatives is similar to that found by Kapur and Pearson [8]. This indicates that the extent of change perceived in memory abilities was much the same for patients and their relatives. However, the correlation between rating scale scores and the memory lapses observed by therapists was much weaker and was not significant, suggesting that both relatives and patients were unaware of the extent of memory impairment following brain injury.

There is virtually no correlation between time postonset and self-rating, which indicates that a person's own view of his or her memory ability is little

Table 8.3   Mean Scores on Rating Scales and Checklists

Source	*Mean*	*SD*	*Range*
Patients' ratings	3.96[a]	3.52	0–13
Relatives' ratings	5.65	3.63	0–13
Therapists' checklists	44.52[b]	58.11	0–289

[a]Maximum was 20.
[b]Maximum was 760.

Table 8.4   Intercorrelational Matrix (Spearman) between Therapist Checklists, Self-Ratings, Relatives' Ratings, and Time Postonset

Checklists	*Self-Ratings*	*Relatives' Ratings*	*Time Postonset*
Checklists —	0.28	0.36	0.44[a]
Self-rating	—	0.83[b]	0.04
Relatives' ratings		—	0.27

[a]$p < 0.05$.
[b]$p < 0.001$.

affected by the length of time since the accident or by whatever influences there may have been during that time. However, in view of the wide differences in length of time between accident and admission to Rivermead, it seemed advisable to explore this in more detail. The subjects could be divided conveniently into two groups: those who had either come straight from the referring acute hospital or had spent a very short time at home and were between 1 and 10 months postonset; and those who had spent considerable time at home before coming to Rivermead and were between 1 and 6 years postonset (Table 8.5).

We looked to see whether there were differences in the following. (1) Self-rating. Do people become more aware of their problems the longer it has been since their accident? (2) Relative rating. Are relatives more aware of a patient's problems when they have been living in close proximity for some time, as distinct from seeing the patient in a hospital setting?

All the differences were nonsignificant. However, there was a trend toward those patients with more recent injury performing better on the Rivermead Behavioral Memory Test (RBMT) (see below) and toward relatives rating patients as worse when they had been living with them longer. If anything, however, patients perceive themselves as less memory impaired the longer the time since the accident. It will be interesting to see if these trends are confirmed with larger numbers. People referred to a rehabilitation center a long time after their accident will generally be those who have considerable residual problems that can no longer be coped with adequately at home without some intervention, whereas those who come during the first few months of recovery are those thought most likely to benefit from early intensive rehabilitation. They are also seen at a stage when they are likely to be making rapid progress.

Patients and relatives agree quite closely on changes in memory performance, although both groups appear to underestimate the extent of decline. It would seem that relatives are slightly more aware of change than patients, and tend to become moreso with the passing of time after the injury. This may be due to growing familiarity with the patient's behavior as observed in everyday settings.

Table 8.5 Scores of Brain-Injured Patients Soon after Injury and Late after Injury

	Short Time Postonset (n = 11)		Long Time Postonset (n = 12)		Mann-Whitney U Test[a]
Source	*(Mean)*	*(SD)*	*(Mean)*	*(SD)*	
Self-rating	4.46	4.08	3.50	3.03	57.5
Relative's rating	2.27	2.97	5.25	5.48	42.0

[a]Differences were not statistically significant.

AUTOBIOGRAPHICAL MEMORY

Until recently, autobiographical memory has not received a great deal of attention. We (Baddeley and Wilson [10]) have reported an attempt to assess and score autobiographical memory in brain-injured subjects. We have also provided a tentative and preliminary taxonomy of autobiographical memory deficit. In our preliminary study we described four patterns of deficit that seemed to be emerging from our observations of 12 amnesic patients. A subgroup of these patients appeared to have access to autobiographical memory, at least for events preceding the onset of amnesia. The second subgroup demonstrated clouded autobiographical memory (they were able to recall certain autobiographical events in some detail on one occasion but not subsequently). The third subgroup (those with marked frontal lobe damage) were able to report extremely little of their earlier lives but showed no evidence of confabulation. This subgroup we described as "dysfluent." Patients in the fourth subgroup, also with marked frontal lobe damage, were fluent but showed considerable confabulation. Members of this subgroup made errors and showed inconsistencies, and also produced bizarre and elaborate stories that were not at all accurate. Examples of each of these subgroups are described in Baddeley and Wilson [10]. Patients with severe brain injury can fall into any one of these categories, illustrating that common etiology does not guarantee similar cognitive dysfunction.

Since the 1986 study [10], we have been collaborating with Michael Kopelman in London in an attempt to produce a systematic autobiographical memory schedule. We ask each subject to describe certain life periods, such as the period before starting school, the first school attended, and so on, until we reach the present day. For each of these time periods, standard questions are asked to elicit information such as, for example, the subject's address at a particular time, the names of three friends, teachers, or colleagues, or important incidents. We are in the process of analyzing information gathered from a range of neurologically impaired people, including a number with severe brain injuries. Preliminary data indicate that brain-injured people are significantly worse than control subjects at remembering details, even from incidents in the distant past, and at remembering facts such as names of past associates.

Autobiographical memory in brain-injured people is potentially important for at least two reasons. First, we have found quite marked differences among patients who are otherwise similar, at least in intelligence quotient (IQ) and memory test scores. Second, we think autobiographical memory might have prognostic importance, for example, in predicting response to treatment. Thus our patients who show gross confabulation seem very likely to be admitted to long-term psychiatric care; those with normal autobiographical memory tend to cope at home despite being densely amnesic. The latter group also seem to be less anxious, agitated, or distressed than those with clouded autobiographical memory. These observations will remain at the most tentative level until further work has been conducted. However, it makes intuitive sense that, to remain intact as individuals, we need to know *who* we are, and that to know this we must have an adequate autobiographical memory.

OTHER TESTS OF REMOTE MEMORY

Butters and Albert [11], in a study of retrograde amnesia suggested that although Korsakoff patients show a temporal gradient in their ability to remember (with earlier memories being better preserved than later ones), patients with Huntington's chorea do not. Relatively little systematic work has focused on retrograde amnesia in brain-injured patients, even though the length of retrograde amnesia has potentially important implications within rehabilitation.

Several assessment procedures have been used to look at remote memory and retrograde amnesia in other groups of patients. These include tests of famous events [12], famous personalities [13], famous faces [14], famous voices [15], and television programs [12]. All of these tests have one or more of the following disadvantages:

1. Problems of overlearning. For example, certain faces or events, such as Charlie Chaplin, or the assassination of President Kennedy, will be so deeply learned that they will be known long after the time period when they were currently famous. Young people are likely to know of such people and events from times before they were born.
2. Differences in exposure time. It is impossible to ensure that all events, personalities, or programs receive the same amount of exposure to the general public.
3. There are large differences in the level of interest of subjects; some take a large interest in current events, but others are almost never aware of news or current affairs.
4. Age differences. Many of the retrograde amnesia tests are designed for use with people of middle or old age. This makes them unsuitable for younger people, because youth and amnesia become confused.
5. These tests are frequently insensitive to short periods of retrograde amnesia (which are common after severe brain injury).
6. Problems with updating. It is time consuming to update retrograde amnesia tests. In addition, it might be difficult to obtain appropriate material.
7. Obtaining the test. Most tests are designed for a specific study or population or diagnostic group, and they are not easy to obtain.

In an attempt to avoid many of these problems, we developed a short test of retrograde amnesia called the "Prices Test" [16]. The test requires people to estimate the current cost of 10 everyday items, for example a first-class stamp, a gallon of gasoline, or a pint of milk. The estimated price is deducted from the actual price and divided by the standard deviation. In effect, something similar to a Z score is obtained. The test was standardized with 100 control subjects who were asked to estimate the cost of 25 items. The 10 items showing least variability were then selected for inclusion in the final version of the test. This has since been given to more than 200 brain-injured people, including 44 with severe brain injury. By totaling the scores for each item, a measure of severity of retrograde amnesia is obtained. An example is given in Table 8.6. We are in the process of plotting out the prices of each item for six-month periods over the past 20 years so that we can estimate the extent of the retrograde amnesia.

It is obvious from this example that it is quite possible to overestimate the cost of items as well as to underestimate them, and indeed some patients with frontal lobe involvement tend to overestimate. Some of the findings from our investigations are reported in Table 8.7.

The main advantages of the Prices Test are the following:

1. It reduces the effect of exposure and learning time.
2. Prices change frequently, so it is more sensitive to short periods of retrograde amnesia than many other retrograde amnesia tests.
3. It is easy to update.
4. It is suitable for a wide range of patients of various ages.

However, like any test, the Prices Test has disadvantages. Certain groups of people such as long-term psychiatric patients are unlikely to be able to do the test. Certain items are less appropriate than others. For example, a portion

Table 8.6   Prices Test[a]

Item	Estimated	Actual	Difference	SD	Score[b]
		Price			
Loaf of bread	12P	45P	−33P	6P	−4
Pint of milk	10P	21P	−11P	2P	−4
New Austin Mini car	£1,000.00	£3,100.00	−£2,100.00	£900.00	−2
20 Rothmans cigarettes	60P	£1.20	−65P	13P	−4
A *Guardian* newspaper	15P	23P	−8P	6P	−1
A gallon of 4-star gasoline	£2.00P	£1.89	−11P	17P	0
1-lb jar of jam	35P	45P	−10P	15P	0
Portion of fish and chips	£1.00	90P	+10P	19P	0
First-class stamp	15P	15P	0	0.5P	0
Cup of coffee on British Rail	14P	35P	−21P	8P	−2

[a]Prices are given in British pounds (£) or pence (P).
[b]Scoring is as follows: ≤ 1 SD, score 0; 1 < SD ≤ 2, score 1; 2 < SD ≤ 3, score 2; 3 < SD ≤ 4, score 4.

Table 8.7 Performance of Diagnostic Groups on the Prices Test

Group	n	Underestimates		Overestimates	
		(Mean)	(SD)	(Mean)	(SD)
Severe brain injury	44	8.40	6.50	3.50	3.40
"Pure" amnesiacs	12	15.66	6.80	1.16	1.53
Non-Korsakoff alcoholics	26	2.50	3.70	3.10	5.10
Elderly normal subjects[a]	12	1.41	2.13	0.60	0.80
Alzheimer-type dementia	9	17.20	6.50	5.70	3.50
Frontal lobe patients (tumor, aneurysm)	7	8.85	5.71	4.14	3.71

[a]Control subjects under the age of 65 years have a mean score of 0 because the test was standardized on this group.

of fish and chips is cheaper in the North of England than in the South, whereas a first-class stamp costs the same throughout the land. It is not easy to use a Prices Test in many other countries. In the United States, for example, prices are much less standardized throughout the country. Finally, it is relatively hard to show a temporal gradient with the Prices Test, because prices of individual items change at different rates. Nevertheless, it is a quick and useful way of determining how "out-of-date" people are. It would be interesting to see research correlating performance on the Prices Test with performance in other areas such as response to rehabilitation, ability to manage financial affairs, and so on.

LEARNING NEW SKILLS

One feature of modern life is that we are expected to learn new technological skills, such as using a computer or manipulating the remote control buttons for a television set. How people learn these skills has not been extensively studied, although we have recently published a study looking at the performance of 100 brain-injured patients and 50 controls when they were required to learn a new technological skill [17]. The particular skill was programming an electronic memory aid. The program consisted of six steps. The instructions and procedure given to each subject were as follows:

"What I am going to do now is to try to teach you to set the date and time on this machine. There are six steps involved: I want you to watch me do it first, and then see if you can do it. Watch what I do."

"The first step is to put this button over to SET." (Put button over.)

"The second step is to put in the month." (Put in month). "For example—it's the third month now, so we put in 03."

"Then we put in the date. It's the 16th (for example), so we put in 16."

"Now we have to tell the machine that that is the date. So we press the DATE button, which is this one here." (Point and press.) "Now we have to put in the time, which is 1:54. So we press 1-5-4.)

"Now we have to tell the machine that that's the time. So we press the TIME button, which is this one here." (Press the TIME button.) "And that's it."

Tester then sets the top button to normal and wipes off previous input by pressing the RESET button on the back.

"Now I'd like you to have a go. What did I do first?"

After each step, any errors are corrected so that each trial eventually succeeds in putting in the appropriate date and time. Subjects are allowed up to three attempts. If all six steps are correct on any one trial, the test stops at that point.

Of the 100 patients, 37 had sustained a severe traumatic brain injury. Findings for this group and for the 50 control subjects are reported in Table 8.8.

Evidence from theoretical studies of memory suggests that procedural learning may be unimpaired in amnesic patients. This might suggest that people with memory impairments have little difficulty in learning new skills, but evidence suggests the contrary. Indeed, we need to ask what is meant by "procedural learning." To define it as skill learning is insufficient. The technological skill reported here correlated significantly with tests of visual, verbal, spatial, and prospective memory. However, the best correlation was with an amalgam of these memory tests, namely, the overall score on the RBMT (a test of everyday memory reported by Wilson et al [18] and described below). Our findings suggest that a technological skill like the one we selected requires a combination of several memory abilities.

THE RBMT

The RBMT [18] was developed to provide an objective test of everyday memory skills that are often affected by acquired brain damage such as a closed head injury. The items were chosen to reflect the problems reported by patients in

Table 8.8 Performance of Brain-Injured and Control Subjects on Learning a New Skill

	Age (yrs)			% Who Learned Task On:			
Subjects	Mean	SD	Range	Trial 1	Trial 2	Trial 3	% Who Failed
Controls (n = 50)	37.3	23.6	16–69	70	28	2	0
Brain-injured (n = 37)	30.9	13.2	14–63	16.2	10.8	16.2	56.7

studies such as those by Sunderland et al [9], and through observation of patients at Rivermead Rehabilitation Centre, Oxford, England.

We wanted a test that would provide practical information relevant to everyday life. Most memory tests have been designed to find out how memory works, not how much individuals are able to do with the memory capacity they possess. Self-report measures were considered but, as we argued in an earlier section, such measures are of limited value despite being quick and having better face validity than many memory tests. In an attempt to combine the objectivity of standardized procedures with the face validity of real-life situations, the RBMT was designed. It had to be a reliable and valid test, not only of memory but also of everyday memory skills.

The test consists of 12 items: remembering a name (this counts as 2 items—first name and surname); remembering to ask for an appointment; remembering to collect a personal belonging; remembering a new route immediately after it has been demonstrated and again after a delay; remembering to deliver a message; picture recognition; face recognition; remembering a newspaper article; remembering the date; and answering orientation questions. There are four parallel versions of the test to reduce practice effects.

To develop and standardize the RBMT, it was given to 175 brain-damaged patients between the ages of 16 and 65 years. Sixty of these had sustained a severe brain injury. Most of the remainder were stroke patients, and a further group had suffered encephalitis, a cerebral tumor, or carbon monoxide poisoning. The test was also administered to 109 control subjects between the ages of 16 and 65 years, and with a mean IQ of 106 (range, 68–136).

The mean score of control subjects was 10.6, with a standard deviation of 1.41 and a range of 7 to 12. The scores of the controls were used to determine cutoff points between normal and abnormal functioning for patients. The mean score of the 60 brain-injured patients was 5.22, with a standard deviation of 3.75 and a range of 0 to 12.

Parallel form reliability was determined by giving two versions of the test to 118 patients. All completed version A, one-third of them also completed version B, another third completed version C, and the final third completed version D. The order of presentation was randomized. Correlation between performance on version A and on versions B,C, and D was 0.84, 0.80, and 0.63, respectively.

Inter-rater reliability was established by having 40 subjects scored separately but simultaneously by two raters. The range of scores was from 0 to 12 (that is, from severely impaired to normal performance). In all, 10 different raters, all psychologists or psychology students, took part in the inter-rater reliability study. There was 100% agreement between the raters.

Validity was established in two ways. First, correlations were determined between performance on the RBMT and scores on other tests of memory. Correlations between RBMT scores and other memory test scores for the brain-injured and stroke patients are reported in Table 8.9 [19–22].

The data appear to indicate that the RBMT is a valid test of memory.

Table 8.9 Correlations between the Rivermead Behavioral Memory Test and Other Tests of Memory

Test (source)	Left CVA[a]	n	Right CVA	n	HI[b]	n	All Patients	n
Recognition memory: words Warrington [19]	0.35	21	0.33	31	0.71	37	0.60	112
Recognition memory: faces Warrington [19]	0.57	23	0.41	32	0.43	40	0.40	119
Digits forward	0.61	24	0.31	39	0.17	42	0.35	135
Digits backward	0.37	24	0.53	38	0.05	42	0.28	134
Paired associate learning Randt et al [20]	0.57	25	0.62	35	0.61	41	0.61	131
Corsi blocks Milner [21]	0.16	24	0.62	38	0.32	46	0.24	139
Semantic processing Baddeley [22]	0.25	23	0.38	35	0.39	42	0.25	129

Abbreviations: CVA = cerebral vascular accident; HI = head injury.

However, we wanted this test to do more than assess memory, per se. Our aim was to assess everyday memory functioning, and we were able to check this out by referring to the direct observations of patients by therapists. In the previous section on self-report measures, we reported that we asked therapists working with the Rivermead patients to complete daily checklists for two weeks. In addition to the 23 brain-injured patients reported on earlier, there were 57 stroke, tumor and encephalitic patients, making a total of 80 brain-damaged people. Correlations between scores on the RBMT and the number of lapses observed by the therapists was highly significant (0.75). Thus, it would seem we have achieved our goal of designing a valid test of everyday memory.

In summary, the RBMT is a short, reliable, valid test of everyday memory problems, is easy to administer and score, and is applicable in a wide range of environmental settings. It can be used as a measure of the severity of memory problems, and as a guide to the selection of treatment goals. It is also acceptable to patients because it has greater face validity than most other memory tests.

CONCLUSION

Severe disablement is frequently experienced by people with memory impairment resulting from brain injury. These people are not helped to achieve more control over their daily lives by the kind of memory assessment that concentrates on performance on unrealistic tasks within the isolated confines of the laboratory or clinic [23]. We prefer those tasks that mirror the kinds of remembering that are required in the routine of daily living. There is a growing realization among psychologists that performance on such tasks can shed light on the kinds of treatment that might be offered to individuals experiencing different kinds and degrees of memory impairment. We have produced valid, reliable forms of assessment that are relatively simple but relate to the real-life needs of memory-impaired people. These include self-report measures, rating scales, checklists, an autobiographical memory schedule, the Prices Test, assessing the learning of new skills, and the RBMT. We believe that these programs represent convincing arguments for the approach we advocate for assessment and treatment of everyday memory functioning following severe brain injury.

REFERENCES

1. Brooks DN. Cognitive deficits. In: Brooks DN, ed. Closed head injury: Psychological, social and family consequences. Oxford: Oxford University Press, 1984.
2. Harris JE, Morris PE, eds. Everyday memory, actions and absentmindedness. London: Academic Press, 1984.

3. Bartram D, Smith P. Everyday memory for everyday places. In: Harris JE, Morris P, eds. Everyday memory, actions and absentmindedness. London: Academic Press, 1984.

4. Harris JE. Remembering to do things: A forgotten topic. In: Harris JE, Morris P, eds. Everyday memory, actions and absentmindedness. London: Academic Press, 1984.

5. Bahrick HP. Memory for people. In: Harris JE, Morris P, eds. Everyday memory, actions and absentmindedness. London: Academic Press, 1984.

6. Sunderland A, Harris JE, Baddeley AD. Do laboratory tests predict everyday memory? A neuropsychological study. J Verbal Learning Verbal Behav 1983;22:341–57.

7. Sunderland A, Harris JE, Gleave J. Memory failures in everyday life after severe head injury. J Clin Neuropsychol 1984;6:127–42.

8. Kapur N, Pearson D. Memory symptoms and memory performance of neurological patients. Br J Psychol 1983;74:409–15.

9. Sunderland A, Harris JE, Baddeley AD. Assessing everyday memory after severe head injury. In: Harris JE, Morris P, eds. Everyday memory, actions and absentmindedness. London: Academic Press, 1984.

10. Baddeley AD, Wilson B. Amnesia, autobiographical memory and confabulation. In: Rubin D, ed. Autobiographical memory. Cambridge: Cambridge University Press, 1986.

11. Butters N, Albert MS. Processes underlying failures to recall remote events. In: Cermak L, ed. Human memory and amnesia. Hillsdale, NJ: Erlbaum, 1982.

12. Squire LR, Cohen NJ. Remote memory, retrograde amnesia and the neuropsychology of memory. In: Cermak L, ed. Human memory and amnesia. Hillsdale, NJ: Erlbaum, 1982.

13. Corkin S, Growden JH, Nissen MJ, Huff FJ, Freed DM, Sagar HJ. Recent advances in the neuropsychological study of Alzheimer's disease. In: Wurtman RJ, Corkin S, Growden JH, eds. Alzheimer's disease: Advances in basic research and therapies. Cambridge MA: Center for Brain Sciences and Metabolism Trust, 1984.

14. Albert MS, Butters N, Levin J. Memory for remote events in chronic alcoholics and Korsakoff patients. In: Begleiter H, Kissen B, eds. Alcohol intoxication and withdrawal. New York: Plenum Press, 1979.

15. Meudell PR, Northen B, Snowden JS, Neary D. Long term memory for famous voices in amnesic and normal subjects. Neuropsychologia 1980;18:133–39.

16. Wilson BA. Identification and remediation of everyday problems in memory impaired adults. In: Nathan P, Butters N, Parsons O, eds. Neuropsychology of alcoholism: Implications for diagnosis and treatment. New York: Guilford Press, 1987.

17. Wilson BA, Cockburn J, Baddeley AD. How do old dogs learn new tricks? Teaching a technological skill to brain injured people. Paper presented to the Annual Conference of the International Neuropsychological Society. Washington, DC, February 1987. (Cortex, in press).

18. Wilson BA, Cockburn J, Baddeley AD. The Rivermead Behavioural Memory Test. Reading, England: Thames Valley Test Co., 1985.

19. Warrington EK. The recognition memory test. Windsor: NFER-Nelson, 1984.

20. Rand CT, Brown ER, Osborne DP. A memory test for longitudinal measurement of mild to moderate deficits. Clin Neuropsychiatry 1980;2:184–94.

21. Milner B. Interhemispheric differences in the localisation of psychological processes in man. Br Med Bull: Cog Psychol 1971;27:272–77.
22. Baddeley AD. The cognitive psychology of everyday life. Br J Exp Psychol 1981;72:257–69.
23. Baddeley AD. Memory theory and memory therapy. In: Wilson B, Moffat N, eds. Clinical management of memory problems. London: Croom Helm, 1984.

Part III

Brain Injury in Children

Michael E. Miner

Trauma is the major cause of death and disability in children and as such it must be a major health concern in this country. Brain injury alone accounts for more deaths in children than acquired immune deficiency syndrome (AIDS), cancer, and congenital disorders combined. However, brain injury in children is different from that in adults in a variety of important ways. Children differ significantly from adults in that they are smaller but are growing and developing. Size in itself is important in how children get injured. The fragility of the child is also related to factors attendant on size, such as blood volume and maintenance of body temperature. Children are supposed to grow. Thus, properly caring for a child means that he or she grows. This brings up the question of nutrition, and there may be important fundamental differences in how children should be nourished compared with adults. However, the most important way that children differ from adults is that children are developing. If an adult returns to baseline function after injury it is viewed as a success. However, if an injured child returns to baseline function and does not develop further, it is a treatment failure. The brain undergoes major changes in physical properties in the first few years of life. The response to injury is also different in children than in adults. Acute cerebral edema following injury is a much more significant problem for infants than for older children. Thus, the intrinsic characteristics of the immature, developing child's brain requires treatment regimens different from that for adults.

During the past few decades it has become evident that children are injured in different ways than adults. Children are more commonly injured in falls and low-velocity injuries. The Hospital for Sick Children in Toronto has made important contributions to the understanding of the demography of brain injury in children. For many years they have maintained records on children's injuries and the outcome of treatment. Robin Humphreys has reported on a six-year experience at that institution. The outcome of their management of brain-injured children reminds us that, although the mortality among severely brain-injured children is high, the outcome in those who survive can be extremely gratifying.

Unfortunately, some of the mechanisms responsible for terrible injuries in adults also occur in children. The treatment of adults with gunshot wounds to the brain is not very gratifying, and the group from the University of Texas in Houston has recounted their experience with guns and children. This type of injury is becoming more common in large urban areas of the United States, and the results are not good. Miner et al have started a community-based educational program aimed toward prevention of these injuries. At this juncture the results are encouraging. However, more to the heart of the issue is how people deal with anger and fear. So long as people try to solve their problems with guns, children will find access to those guns and be injured.

Monitoring of brain-injured children may be different from that of adults. James Hall et al have used electrical parameters to monitor brain-injured children in the intensive care setting. They have found that monitoring of evoked potentials is useful in evaluating therapy in the severely injured, and have discovered a technique that extends the ability to evaluate comatose children.

One of the more difficult questions in brain-injured children is: how does one evaluate outcome? There are unique problems in children that make it vital to evaluate their cognitive skills. Jack Fletcher et al recount their extensive experience in monitoring cognitive outcome after brain injury in children. Such information is especially important because school systems can use data such as these to develop special programs to help. It must be remembered that the public school system in the United States provides both therapy and education for brain-injured children. Fletcher et al also describe which tools are particularly valuable in evaluating cognitive congenital or perinatal disorders of neurologic function. Systems that are built to support those children will need some modification before they can benefit brain-injured children.

Chapter 9

Adaptive Behavior in Brain-Injured Children

Jack M. Fletcher
Linda Ewing-Cobbs
Michael E. Miner
Harvey S. Levin
Howard M. Eisenberg

The neuropsychological and behavioral sequelae of pediatric closed head injury are the subject of numerous recent studies [1,2]. Although the precise nature and long-term course of these sequelae are not well understood, it has been established that brain injury in children is associated with major residual difficulties in (1) measures of performance-based intelligence [3]; (2) speeded motor abilities [4]; (3) memory and attention [5]; and (4) behavioral adjustment [6]. Of these sequelae, changes in the child's behavior and adaptive functioning at home and at school have been studied infrequently. The absence of research is unfortunate because behavioral problems are frequent concerns of parents and teachers, particularly in the period from three months to three years postinjury. This period occurs after many of the major physical effects of the trauma have been stabilized, and represents a time at which most injured children are home from the hospital and have returned to school. During this time, the child seems different to parents and may be more difficult to manage at home and at school. The success of various therapies addressing cognitive and motor disabilities after pediatric brain injury may depend on how well the child re-adapts to home and school. Hence, residual difficulties in behavioral adjustment may be important determinants of the child's long-term recovery.

The purpose of this chapter is to discuss the behavioral sequelae of pediatric brain injury. After a review of relevant studies, including data from our own follow-up of brain-injured children, factors in the assessment and management of behavioral problems after pediatric brain injury will be presented.

BEHAVIOR AFTER BRAIN INJURY IN CHILDREN

The study of behavioral problems after brain injury in children has been influenced by traditional conceptions of the relationship of brain injury and behavioral change. Many practitioners believe that brain injury in children leads to a characteristic, unitary behavioral pattern. This pattern is characterized by behavior that is overactive, impulsive, and distractible. Although the origins of this conception date back to the beginning of this century [7], the most significant influence has stemmed from the work of Straus and Lehtinen [8]. Based on observations of mentally retarded children, these authors argued that certain forms of mental retardation reflected "minimal brain injury" characterized by perseveration, impulsivity, behavioral overactivity, concreteness in thinking, and emotional lability. This behavioral pattern was assumed to be a unitary consequence of brain injury. Observation of these behaviors in children without objective neurological evidence of brain impairment was regarded as sufficient to justify an inference of central nervous system (CNS) dysfunction. Based on this argument, terms such as *minimal brain damage* as well as numerous hypotheses concerning appropriate methods of treating the *brain-injured* child were derived [7,9].

The problems with these conceptions have been widely described [2,7,10]. There is little evidence supporting the presence of a unitary behavioral disorder after various forms of brain injury in children. In fact, behavioral outcomes after brain injury in children are diverse, and are influenced by a number of environmental variables [6,11]. Given the diversity of CNS pathology in children, this finding is hardly surprising. Even within diagnoses such as brain injury, behavioral outcomes vary widely, depending on the nature of the injury and the environment. Some brain-injured children are impulsive and overactive, whereas others are more quiet and withdrawn. Certain children may demonstrate both patterns at different points during recovery. Hence, attributing unitary forms of behavior problems to brain injury is simplistic and inconsistent with current outcome data.

BEHAVIORAL CHANGES AFTER PEDIATRIC BRAIN INJURY

The multidetermined nature of behavioral change after brain injury is clearly apparent in studies of recovery in children. Early studies were poorly controlled. For example, Blau [12] suggested that brain injuries were associated with generally disinhibited behavior. However, many of these patients were still in early phases of recovery. Black et al found that only 20% of brain-injured children, most of whom sustained mild injuries, showed behavioral problems one year postinjury [13].

English Study

The most systematic studies of posttraumatic behavioral disturbances were completed in England [6,11]. Brown et al [6] found that the severity of brain injury was related to the likelihood of behavioral difficulties. However, other factors, including the child's premorbid characteristics and the postinjury environment, were also contributory, particularly in milder injuries.

The English study divided children into mild and severe brain injury groups according to the length of posttraumatic amnesia (PTA). PTA is commonly defined as the interval during which confusion and anterograde amnesia (i.e., inability to consolidate information about ongoing events) are present after emergence from coma. In severe cases, PTA persisted for at least one week; in mild cases PTA persisted from 1 hour to less than 7 days. The brain-injured groups were matched on a variety of social and demographic variables with a group of children who had sustained orthopedic injuries. Parent and teacher interviews and personality questionnaires were administered at the time of injury and at 4 months, 1 year, and more than 2 years postinjury. The mild injury group had a higher rate of preinjury behavioral disturbance than either the severe injury or control groups. This implies that children who sustained mild injuries were behaviorally different before the injury. Such a finding is consistent with the hypotheses that children who are impulsive and active are more likely to take the kinds of risks that lead to brain injury. In contrast, the severe injury group did not show a raised frequency of preinjury behavioral disturbances relative to controls.

The relationship between severity of injury and psychiatric disorders arising after the injury is depicted in Figure 9.1.

No differences in the rate of new disorders were observed between the mild injury and control groups on any of the follow-up assessments (see Figure 9.1). In contrast, in approximately half of the severe brain injury group, new psychiatric disorders developed. By 27 months postinjury, the rate of behavioral disturbance was three times higher in the severe injury group than in the control group. Although mild brain injury was not associated with an increased incidence of disturbance, severe brain injury was clearly associated with a marked increase in the rate of psychiatric disorder. Behavioral problems commonly reflected preinjury behavior such that preexisting difficulties were exacerbated after injury. Similarly, adverse social circumstances in the preinjury environment were also related to the presence of behavioral disturbances after severe brain injury. Rutter et al [6,11] also found that there was a weak relationship between the degree of cognitive disturbance and postinjury behavioral sequelae.

Houston/Galveston Study

Our group is currently evaluating cognitive and behavioral functioning at the time of injury and 6, 12, 24, and 36 months postinjury in brain-injured children

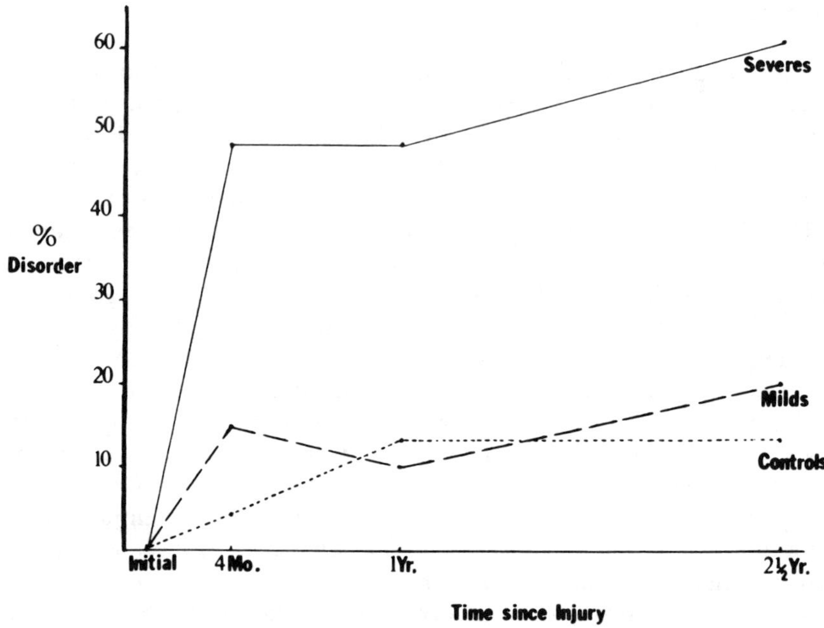

Figure 9.1   Rates of new psychiatric disorders following head injury in children. Reprinted with permission of the author and publisher.

aged 0 through 15 years. These children were recruited from the University Children's Hospital at Hermann and John Sealy Hospital after admission for traumatic brain injury. The initial evaluation occurred after resolution of PTA as measured by the Children's Orientation and Amnesia Test (COAT [14]). The COAT is an objective, normed measure of orientation and memory developed by Harvey S. Levin and other members of our group.

Children were placed into two groups based on a combination of Glasgow Coma Score (GCS) [15], duration of impaired consciousness, and results of CT scans. The duration of impaired consciousness was defined as the number of days a child was unable to follow one-stage commands such as "squeeze my hand." Children with severe brain injuries (n = 16) had GCS values on hospital admission ranging from 3 to 12; all children exhibited impaired consciousness for at least 24 hours. Mild/moderate brain injury (n = 26) was defined by GCS values ranging from 9 to 15 and impaired consciousness persisting for less than 24 hours. CT scan abnormalities may have been present in children with moderate traumatic brain injury (TBI).

Table 9.1 presents demographic characteristics of the mild/moderate and severe TBI groups. As Table 9.1 shows, the groups were entirely comparable in age, gender, ethnicity, and socioeconomic status. Neurologic indexes of severity of injury are contained in Table 9.2. GCS values and the duration of

Table 9.1 Demographic Characteristics of Brain-Injured Children

Variable	Injury Severity	
	Mild/Moderate *(n = 26)*	*Severe* *(n = 16)*
Age (mo)		
$\bar{x}$	78.1	102.5
SD	59.2	51.6
Socioeconomic status[a]		
Low	17	6
Middle	5	7
High	4	3
Gender		
Male	13	10
Female	13	6
Ethnicity		
Black	6	7
White	18	3
Hispanic	3	6

[a]Based on the Hollingshead Two-Factor Index of Social Position.

impaired consciousness clearly differentiated the mild/moderate from the severe TBI groups. Severely injured children were comatose for an average of 7.7 days.

To evaluate the impact of TBI on social and behavioral functioning, the Child Behavior Checklist (CBCL) [16] and the Vineland Adaptive Behavior Scales (VABS) [17] were completed by one parent from each family. These measures were administered as soon after the injury as possible to obtain a comparatively unbiased estimate of the child's level of functioning before the injury. The CBCL and VABS were readministered 6 and 12 months postinjury to characterize changes in psychiatric symptoms and adaptive behavior.

The CBCL is a well-known behavioral rating scale for children 4 to 16 years of age. The parent completes items pertaining to social competency and possible behavior problems. Items addressing behavior problems are scored on a scale from 0 to 2, with 0 representing no problems and 2 representing a frequent or significant problem for the child. Extensive factor analytic and reliability studies have led to the creation of a set of eight or nine basic scales (depending on the child's age) sensitive to disordered behavior (e.g., depressed,

Table 9.2 Neurologic Characteristics of Brain-Injured
Children

	Injury Severity	
Variable	*Mild/Moderate* *(n = 26)*	*Severe* *(n = 16)*
No. of children with GCS of:		
3–8	0	12
9–12	1	4[a]
13–15	25	0
Days of impaired consciousness		
$\bar{x}$	0.05	7.72
SD	0.15	7.15
Range	0–0.5	1.5–31.0
No. of children injured by:		
Motor vehicle	8	5
Motor vehicle– pedestrian accident	2	9
Fall	15	1
Other	1	1

[a]Although four severely injured children had acute Glasgow Coma
Scores (GCS) of 9 through 12, they were classified as having
severe injuries due to deterioration or inability to follow commands for 24 hours.

aggressive, hyperactive). Although the CBCL yields a variety of scales, for the
purposes of this study, scores for internalizing and externalizing factors were
examined. In addition, activities, social, and school scales are presented from
the social competency area. These factors are invariant across age. Because
the other specific scale factors vary with age, interpretation is difficult in a
longitudinal study.

One parent (usually the mother) was also interviewed to complete the
VABS. These scales yield an overall composite score for adaptive functioning
and separate scores for communication, daily living, and socialization domains.
This scale is a revision and restandardization of the Vineland Social Maturity
Scale. Items in each domain are scored from 0 to 2 by the examiner based on
the degree to which the behavior is habitually demonstrated by the child. The
scale was standardized on a national sample of about 3,000 children from birth
to 19 years of age.

Figures 9.2 and 9.3 summarize results for the internalizing and externalizing factors on the CBCL. As these figures show, children with both severe

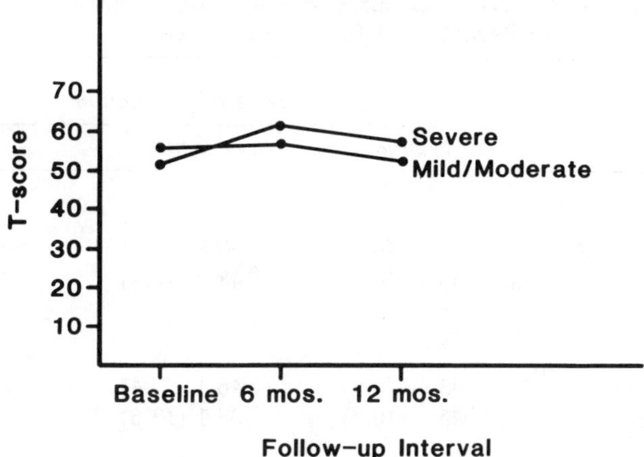

Figure 9.2   Internalizing scores from the Child Behavior Checklist.

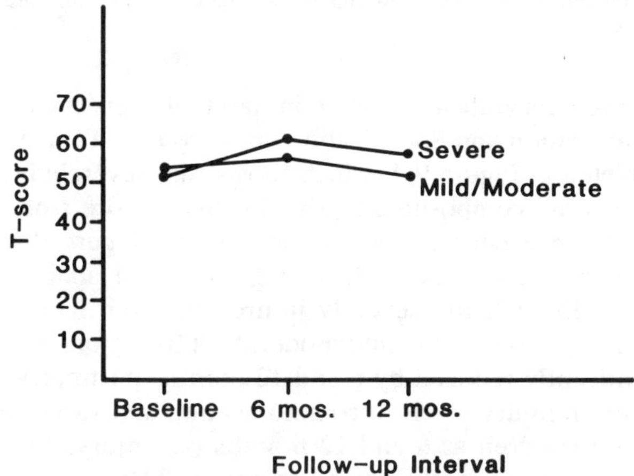

Figure 9.3   Externalizing scores from the Child Behavior Checklist.

and mild/moderate injuries scored within average levels at baseline and showed no changes over time. Group differences were not statistically significant. Similarly, as Table 9.3 shows, no group differences or changes over time were apparent on social or activities scales. However, at 6 months postinjury, parents indicated that severely injured children had more school problems than those sustaining mild/moderate injuries. This difference persisted at 12 months post-injury.

In contrast to the largely null findings from the CBCL, severely injured

Table 9.3 Child Behavior Checklist Social Competence Scores
According to Injury Severity and Time of Evaluation[a]

| | Time of Evaluation | | |
Variable	Preinjury	6 mo	12 mo
Activities			
Mild/moderate	47.1 (6.1)	50.8 (3.4)	50.0 (6.4)
Severe	45.1 (10.6)	48.2 (8.8)	44.8 (8.8)
Social			
Mild/moderate	43.4 (6.9)	46.1 (7.4)	46.5 (8.9)
Severe	45.8 (10.3)	38.1 (13.6)	43.3 (9.0)
School			
Mild/moderate	47.9 (7.3)	45.4 (11.5)	41.1 (10.1)
Severe	44.3 (7.0)	29.7 (12.6)	35.2 (14.6)

[a]Values are standard t scores ($\bar{x}$ = 50, SD = 10). Standard deviations are indicated in parentheses.

children experienced a significant decline in habitual everyday activities on the Vineland Communication and Socialization domains (see Table 9.4). This clear difference is depicted in Figure 9.4, which shows that severely injured children declined on the overall composite adaptive behavior score from baseline to 6 months. This difference persisted at 12 months. As Figure 9.4 shows, mild/moderate injuries are associated with average levels of adaptive behavior at each time point. Although the severely injured children had only somewhat lower scores than children with mild/moderate TBI before the injury, their scores were significantly reduced by 6 and 12 months postinjury. Performance was reduced from preinjury levels in communication and socialization domains in severely injured children at 6 and 12 months postinjury. In contrast, daily living skills were not significantly altered by severe TBI.

The VABS results clearly show that the severely injured children decline in their capacity to perform everyday, habitual communication and socialization behaviors. This decline was not detected by the CBCL, which does not seem to be as sensitive to the behavioral changes characteristic of severely brain-injured children. This may reflect the interview-based format of the VABS, which allows parents to talk more freely about the difficulties experienced by the child. The CBCL items are not specific to brain injury or even to neurological populations in general, which may limit their sensitivity.

Our preliminary results are also somewhat different from those of the English studies. We did not find a higher incidence of behavioral problems in the mild injury group at baseline. This discrepancy may reflect sampling and classification differences. The "mild" patients in the English studies were

Table 9.4 Performance on the Vineland Adaptive Behavior Domains by Injury Severity and Time of Evaluation[a]

	Time of Evaluation		
Domain	*Preinjury*	*6 mo*	*12 mo*
Communication			
Mild/moderate	97.7 (14.9)	97.0 (11.4)	96.1 (11.7)
Severe	86.4 (10.8)	76.5 (15.2)	80.9 (17.5)
Daily living			
Mild/moderate	98.9 (14.3)	100.5 (13.8)	101.7 (11.1)
Severe	89.4 (12.8)	84.8 (10.8)	85.9 (17.2)
Socialization			
Mild/moderate	97.8 (12.2)	96.9 (11.7)	95.7 (11.7)
Severe	90.9 (11.6)	81.1 (15.9)	83.4 (12.8)

[a]Values are standard scores ($\bar{x} = 100$, SD $= 15$). Standard deviations are given in parentheses.

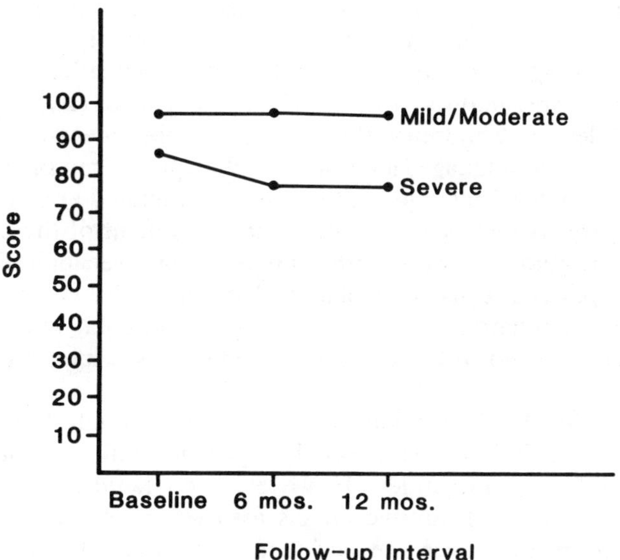

Figure 9.4   Longitudinal performance on the Vineland Adaptive Behavior Scales composite score according to severity of injury.

probably more severely injured than our patients, because PTA could range up to 7 days. However, such a patient would likely be classified as "moderate" in our study. This explanation is limited because mild/moderate injuries received comparable scores on the CBCL and VABS throughout the follow-up period. Additional investigation of this problem with a larger sample is needed to determine whether our "moderates" and "milds" are different on these variables.

Regardless of the interpretation of the results, both our study and the English study show that behavioral adjustment is reduced in children with severe brain injuries. The question, of course, is what to do about this problem area. Simply referring the child for behavior management or psychotherapeutic intervention is not sufficient. Indeed, changes in behavior must be dealt with in the larger context of the child's habilitation.

ASSESSMENT AND MANAGEMENT

The successful habilitation of the brain-injured child requires systematic follow-up, including repeat neuropsychological assessment, liaison with schools and parents, and careful attention to the child's behavior in the context of the family and school placement. Our approach to case management begins in the hospital immediately after injury. An interdisciplinary team evaluates the child's cognitive and behavioral capacities throughout the recovery period, including quantification of PTA with instruments such as the COAT.

When a sufficient level of orientation and working memory is apparent from the COAT, a baseline neuropsychological evaluation is obtained that supplements ongoing work with speech therapy, occupational therapy, and other disciplines. This battery consists of an intelligence (IQ) test (Wechsler Intelligence Scales for Children—Revised) and achievement tests, along with standard measures of language, memory, tactile, spatial, motor, and constructional skills [18]. After discharge, children are reevaluated at 6, 12, 24, and 36 months postinjury. After each evaluation, an assessment of the child's educational progress is made. Liaisons with schools, private rehabilitation agencies, and other disciplines are used to plan and evaluate the child's remediation program. Recommendations for special classes, curricula, and other similar needs are communicated to the parents and educators responsible for treating the child.

We assess the child's behavior at home and at school. The need for this careful monitoring of behavior is especially apparent in children with preexisting behavioral and family difficulties. However, even families that were intact before injury can suffer disruptive effects associated with the trauma. These effects range from guilt over the accident to altered relationships between siblings. General feelings of resentment may be directed toward the injured child because of the amount of care required. School personnel frequently require explanations not only of the child's strengths and weaknesses, but also of the nature of the brain injury and its consequences for behavior. When problems arise and short-term solutions are not applicable, referrals for counseling and pharmacological intervention are considered. School-based interventions emphasize the appropriateness of classroom placement, the need for special services, and appropriate expectations for the injured child.

CONCLUSIONS

Children with severe brain injuries are at risk for cognitive and behavioral difficulties that can persist for several years. Outcomes following injury are heterogeneous, and no single remediation strategy is optimal for every child. Our goal is careful assessment and systematic case management over time. As members of one discipline among many, psychologists provide relatively little direct treatment. However, liaisons with schools, parents and remediation agents can affect the child's postinjury behavior. Hopefully, this kind of systematic, long-term follow-up will facilitate the child's readjustment in the family and at school.

ACKNOWLEDGMENT

Supported in part by funds from the NIH Grant NS-21889, Neurobehavioral Outcome of Head Injury in Children.

REFERENCES

1. Fletcher JM, Levin HS. Neurobehavioral effects of brain injury in children. In: Routh D, ed. Handbook of pediatric psychology. New York: Guilford, 1988;258–95.
2. Oddy M. Head injury during childhood: The psychological implication. In: Brooks DN, ed. Closed head injury: Psychological, social, and family consequences. Oxford: Oxford University Press, 1984;179–94.
3. Winogron HW, Knights RM, Bawden HN. Neuropsychological deficits following head injury in children. J Clin Neuropsychol 1984;66:269–86.
4. Bawden HN, Knights RM, Winogron HW. Speeded performance following head injury in children. J Clin Neuropsychol 1985;7:39–54.
5. Levin HS, Eisenberg HM, Wigg NR, Kobayashi K. Memory and intellectual ability after head injury in children and adolescents. Neurosurgery 1982;11:668–73.
6. Brown G, Chadwick O, Shaffer D, Rutter M, Traub M. A prospective study of children with head injuries. III. Psychiatric sequelae. Psychol Med 1982;11:63–78.
7. Rutter M. Psychological sequelae of brain damage in children. Am J Psychiatry 1984;138:1533–44.
8. Straus AA, Lehtinen LE. Psychopathology and education of the brain injured child. Orlando, FL: Grune & Stratton, 1947.

9. Satz P, Fletcher JM. Minimal brain dysfunction: An appraisal of current research concepts and methods. In: Rie H, Rie E, eds. Handbook of minimal brain dysfunctions. New York: John Wiley, 1980;669–715.
10. Fletcher JM, Taylor HG. Neuropsychological approaches to children: Towards a developmental neuropsychology. J Clin Neuropsychol 1984;6:39–56.
11. Rutter M. Developmental neuropsychiatry: Concepts, issues, and problems. J Clin Neuropsychol 1982;4:91–115.
12. Blau A. Mental changes following head trauma in children. Arch Neurol Psychiatry 1936;35:733–69.
13. Black P, Blumer D, Wellner AM, Walker AE. The head injured child: Time course of recovery with implications for recovery. Proceedings of an International Conference on Head Injury. Edinburgh: Churchill Livingstone, 1972;131–37.
14. Ewing-Cobbs L, Levin HS, Fletcher JM, McLaughlin EJ, McNeely D, Ewert J, Francis D. Assessment of posttraumatic amnesia in head injured children. Paper presented at the meeting of the International Neuropsychological Society, Houston, TX, 1984.
15. Teasdale G, Jennett B. Assessment of coma and impaired consciousness: A practical scale. Lancet 1974;2:81–84.
16. Achenbach TM, Edelbrook C. Manual for the Child Behavior Checklist. New York: Queen City Printers, 1982.
17. Sparrow S, Balla D, Cichetti D. Vineland Adaptive Behavior Scales. Circle Pines, MN: American Guidance Services, 1984.
18. Fletcher JM. Brain-injured children. In: Mash E, Terdal L, eds. Behavioral assessment of childhood disorders. New York: Guilford, 1988;451–89.

Chapter 10

Patterns of Pediatric Brain Injury

Robin P. Humphreys

Virtually all children, at one time or another, sustain brain trauma of varying severity. The galaxy of injuries producing craniocerebral insults is staggering. A gentle tumble from a low-lying sofa cushion to a thickly carpeted floor may result in a widely diastased skull fracture in a six-month-old infant, whereas the cerebral violence associated with a gunshot wound to the head is quite akin to similar injuries in adults. Between these extremes, children sustain brain injuries by falling out of or down from, ejecting through, passing in front of, or being struck by a variety of environmental objects. Their reaction to injury also varies, for children may become acutely ill quite quickly but may also improve with equal rapidity. Fortunately, their ill-defined "biologic plasticity" usually works toward completeness of recovery.

MINOR BRAIN INJURY

The great majority of children with minor brain injuries follow a characteristic clinical pattern. Unconsciousness may or may not have followed the insult. Regardless, the child is irritable, lethargic, and pyrexic, and usually experiences repeated episodes of profuse vomiting. The latter is particularly alarming to parents. It is the persisting, distressing nature of these symptoms that brings the child to the emergency room for assessment and, usually, hospitalization. It is because of these symptoms, or loss of consciousness (known or strongly suspected), or linear skull fractures that hospitals have the policy of admitting children for a minimum observation period of 24 hours. The treatment is symptomatic only and, as a rule, the child will revert to normal within 24 to 48 hours of injury.

The vast majority of children's brain injuries follow such an uneventful course. In his original review from the Hospital for Sick Children (HSC) in Toronto, Hendrick found that only 7% of 4,465 brain-injured children had suffered injuries "severe" enough to require early operative care [1]. In the present study, 5.8% of 3,256 children admitted with brain injury were classified as having "severe" damage according to current definitions. This group of children is the subject of this review.

CLINICAL MATERIAL

The management program of 189 severely brain-injured children consecutively admitted to the intensive care unit (ICU) at HSC between 1 January 1979 and 30 June 1985 have been reviewed. Children admitted to the ICU who had major injuries in other body systems as well as minor brain trauma have been excluded from the review. The children ranged in age from 1 week to 19 years (mean, 7.5 years). Traffic accidents or falls were responsible for 89% of the injuries (Table 10.1). The first HSC neurosurgical review was performed within 6 hours in 153 children, and all but 16 were assessed within 12 hours of trauma.

Immediately upon arrival at HSC, whether the child was sent directly to the ICU or first to the emergency room, standard resuscitation and stabilization measures were begun, and the patient's treatment program followed the algorithm previously outlined [2,3]. The Glasgow Coma Score (GCS) was calculated for all patients still in coma 6 hours later [4]. If it had not been instituted before arrival, orotracheal or nasotracheal intubation was established. Hypovolemic shock, when present, was treated appropriately, but in 8 children, a combination of that and severe brain trauma caused early death (within 24 hours). Patients with other major system injuries that predominated over the brain injury were excluded from the study. Thus, the neurosurgical treatment

Table 10.1 Severe Brain Injury: Causation

Cause	*No. of Patients*
Motor vehicle accident	
Pedestrian/cyclist	96
Passenger	49
Fall	24
Abuse	12
Miscellaneous	
Missile	4
Boating	1
Aircraft	1
Falling tree	1
"Blow"	1

plan was initiated in those children in whom the brain injury was the major insult. CT brain scans were obtained in 162 patients.

Once the patient's initial condition was stabilized, continued intensive care was provided by full-time intensive care specialists working in conjunction with the neurosurgical staff. Intracranial pressure (ICP) was monitored in 108 children. Hyperventilation maintained ICP below 20 torr, arterial carbon dioxide tension ($PaCO_2$) between 25 and 30 torr, arterial oxygen tension (PaO_2) between 150 and 200 torr. When escalations in ICP occurred, manual ventilation was begun, thiopentone was initiated in a push dose of 5 mg/kg, and maintenance therapy was established at 5 to 10 mg/kg per hour. If barbiturate coma was required for control of ICP, phenobarbital was given in a push dose of 30 to 40 mg/kg with maintenance of 20 to 30 mg/kg per day. Muscle paralysis was effected with pancuronium, (0.15 mg/kg push, and 0.1 mg/kg per hour). During this study, there was less reliance than usual upon the ad hoc administration of mannitol and decompressive craniectomy to provide relief from increased ICP.

The follow-up in this series varies from 6 months to 7 years. Of the 189 children in this study, 77 died from their brain injury. The degree of recovery of the 112 survivors is scaled according to the criteria of Jennett and Bond [5]. A further modification into group I (good recovery and moderately disabled), group II (severely disabled and vegetative), and dead, allowed comparison of the HSC results with those published earlier from the Children's Hospital of Philadelphia (Table 10.2) [6].

RESULTS

In this report, the entry features of the patients in the HSC study are itemized to compare the children studied with those in an earlier report by Bruce et al

Table 10.2 Comparison of Severe Brain Injuries: Entry Features

Feature	
No. of patients	189
Average age (yrs)	7.5
Lucid interval (%)	17
Mass lesion (%)	32
Decerebrate/flaccid (%)	56
Hemiparesis (%)	31
Bilateral fixed pupils (%)	35
Mortality (%)	41

[6]. The GCS was calculated for all patients 6 hours or more after trauma; it is stressed again that our review considers only those children with a GCS of 7 or less (Table 10.3).

Although early CT scans were not a mandatory criterion for a child's admission to the study, 162 patients had at least one such examination. The most common abnormality on the scans was diffuse cerebral swelling (66 patients) [7]. Such a finding is an indicator of poor outcome: 32 of these patients are dead, and 25 are disabled. Of the 27 children who were not scanned, 9 had surface clots diagnosed by bedside techniques and were operated on immediately, as were 2 children with compound wounds. Fourteen other children were in extremis, and resuscitative efforts precluded CT assessment. All 14 children died within a few hours of admission.

ICP monitoring, usually with a subarachnoid bolt, was used in 108 children, particularly those who were to be treated with pancuronium paralysis and therapeutic barbiturate coma (Table 10.4). ICP monitoring was not used in many infants, in children with extensive skull fracturing and subgaleal bleeding, or in patients in whom intracranial hematoma had been removed or skull decompressions had been performed. There was no reliable correlation between ICP levels and outcome (Table 10.5). Twenty-eight deaths occurred in children whose ICP, when measured, was greater than 20 torr. However, there were 10 patients who perished and whose ICP was consistently less than 20 torr. Seven of those children were agonal during their several hours of monitoring.

Table 10.3 Severe Brain Injury: Glasgow Coma Score (GCS) at Entry

GCS	No. of Patients
3, 4	85
5–7	104

Table 10.4 Severe Brain Injury: Intracranial Pressure (ICP) and Glasgow Coma Score (GCS)

| | No. of Patients | |
ICP (torr)	GCS = 3, 4	GCS = 5–7
20	19	35
20–30	15	14
>30	16	9

Table 10.5   Severe Brain Injury: Glasgow Coma Score (GCS) and Outcome

	Outcome		
GCS	Group I[a]	Group II[b]	Dead
3, 4	9	18	59
5–7	65	20	18
	39%	20%	41%

[a]Good recovery and moderately disabled.
[b]Severely disabled and vegetative.

DISCUSSION

Each year in North America, brain injury claims the lives of 13,200 young people (less than 19 years of age) [8]. In children 0 to 14 years old, brain trauma is the preeminent cause of death, proving five times more lethal than leukemia, the next most common cause of pediatric mortality [8,9]. These observations are small comfort for those who believe that children make a better recovery than adults after suffering severe brain injury. Previous studies on this subject have suggested that such might be true, as the reported mortality rates in children with "severe" brain injury varied from 6% to 21% [6,9,10].

The purpose of this review is to analyze the treatment results in 189 severely brain-injured children from the HSC, which is a large urban tertiary care facility that receives injured patients directly from the scene of trauma as well as from other primary and secondary care hospitals. In addition to access to major road transport systems, the hospital has a rooftop heliport for helicopter air ambulance landing. Children who died within 6 hours of trauma have been excluded from this series, but the 13 patients who died within 12 hours of injury have been included because they were still being evaluated and resuscitated 6 hours after trauma. Although 6 hours does not, as Jennett and Teasdale state, "represent a time interval of crucial biological significance, it does provide an interval during which initial resuscitation can be completed," [11]. We have thus adhered to their rule of excluding patients who died or became brain dead during this period, as their prognosis was no longer in doubt.

Triage, GCS, and the Child

Two areas of difficulty were encountered with regard to the examination of records on patients deemed to have "severe" brain trauma [12]. Both of these features related to the GCS, which has proven to be the most reliable predictor of outcome. Jennett and Teasdale recommended restricting the definition of severe brain injury to patients who cannot open their eyes, respond verbally, or obey commands for a period of 6 hours or more after injury or deterioration [11]. This is equivalent to a GCS of 7 (or less). A criticism of the latter scale is that it may not be applicable to children less than 3 years of age, whose speech maturation may prohibit interpretation of the examiner's verbal commands. However, this potential restriction is inapplicable to children with "severe" brain trauma; by definition, their GCS could be as high as 9 (eyes: 2 + motor: 5 + verbal: 2) and not require any verbal skills. Moreover, it may be that the motor scale alone is the best indicator of outcome in children.

The second observation challenged the assumption that any patient admitted to an ICU with a brain injury automatically had a "severe" injury and thereby would have a GCS of 7 or less. Such was not the case. The ICU transport team may have admitted the patient via air ambulance to their unit and contacted neurosurgical personnel after the patient's condition was stabilized. The central location of the ICU facilitates triage by multiple on-site specialists. Also, there were several children, especially those with early posttraumatic seizures, whose altered neurological function appeared worse than it was and who required several hours of assessment before their condition dramatically improved. Finally, children who are inappropriately sedated or pharmacologically paralyzed as the result of ambitious care in a primary hospital have been admitted to the ICU until the effects of drug paralysis subside. The induced paralysis masks the initial neurological examination, which may still be obscured at 6 hours posttrauma.

Etiological Factors

Falls are the commonest cause of brain trauma in children, accounting for 53% of all such injuries regardless of severity [1]. However, given the definition of "severe brain injury," traffic accidents account for 77% (145/189) of all children so injured; 96 children were struck as pedestrians or cyclists by automobiles. Forty-nine children were injured as passengers within automobiles, and many were hurled from the vehicle at the moment of impact.

Twenty-four children were injured as the result of falls. The distance varied from off a low couch to up to ten stories via an open apartment window or balcony. Some of the younger children were harmed by tumbling downstairs while in an infant walker.

Age and Outcome

The factors strongly related to outcome and severe brain injuries have been identified as patient age, aspects of coma, autonomic abnormalities, and intracranial hematoma [11,13]. It is commonly stated that children make a better recovery than adults after severe brain injury. Jennett and Teasdale [11] believe that "age has an effect on outcome that is independent of the state of coma, eye movements and pupil reactions, but its effect is less apparent in the most severely injured patients (who do badly whatever their age)." They reported a 35% mortality following severe brain trauma in patients 5 to 19 years of age, and Becker et al [14] found a 22% mortality in patients 0 to 20 years old. Bruce et al [6] have addressed the problem of age and severe brain injury; they report a mortality rate of 6%, which contrasts markedly with the much higher rate quoted in reports dealing predominantly with adults. In the Data Bank Series, children less than 5 years old had a higher mortality than those 5 to 19 years old [11]. Berger et al [15] and Bruce et al [6], on the contrary, found no relationship between age of child and outcome. In the HSC review, children less than 5 years of age represented 38% of the patients but accounted for 61% (47/77) of the deaths, and this subset in a pediatric review suggests that age *is* a reliable indicator of outcome.

GCS and Outcome

The initial GCS is a reliable predictor of outcome (Table 10.5). Fifty-nine of 77 deaths occurred in patients with a GCS of 3 or 4, and of the 27 survivors in this GCS category, 18 are severely disabled or vegetative. Only 9 children are considered normal or moderately disabled. Thus, a child who presents at 6 hours posttrauma with a GCS of 3 or 4 has a 69% risk of mortality, a 21% chance of recovery to severe disability or vegetative condition, and a 10% chance of recovering to normal or to moderate disability. In 103 children with an initial GCS of 5, 6, or 7, 18 are dead, 20 are severely disabled or vegetative, and 65 are normal or moderately disabled. We did not find, as did Bruce et al [16], that a "Glasgow Coma Scale of 5 or greater was always associated with an excellent recovery." At best, 63% of the children in our series could anticipate recovery to the normal or moderately disabled categories.

ICP and Outcome

There was no reliable correlation between ICP levels and outcome (Table 10.6). Although the numbers are small, they are at variance with the accepted principle that mortality rate is related to the presence and degree of increased ICP. Bruce et al [16] report a mortality of 9% in 85 children studied; Langfitt and Gennarelli [17], in a review of 140 children, stated that their mortality was 11% and that none of the children who died had ICP recordings less than 40 torr. Similarly, Berger et al note that patients whose ICP remained greater than 40 torr "either died or left with severe deficits" [15]. In the HSC series, 10 children who had normal ICP died, presumably from brain stem disruption

Table 10.6   Severe Brain Injury: Intracranial Pressure (ICP) and Outcome

ICP	No. of Patients		
(torr)	Group I[a]	Group II[b]	Dead
0–20	27	15	10
20–30	7	13	10
>30	6	2	18

[a]Good recovery and moderately disabled.
[b]Severely disabled and vegetative.

or high cervical cord damage. In 10 other children, ICP levels were less than 30 torr before death. Paradoxically, 6 children with ICP recorded at 30 torr or greater had a group I recovery. These observations might support the opinion of Narayan et al that ICP data were ineffective as the sole indicator of outcome [18].

HSC Outcome

The categories we used to describe recovery in children's severe brain injuries are those used in other series—good, moderately disabled, severely disabled, vegetative, and dead. In order to match the recovery states with those described by Bruce et al [6], only three groupings have been used (Table 10.7). In this series, only 18% (34/189) of children with severe brain injury made a recovery

Table 10.7   Severe Brain Injury: Outcome in 189 Patients

Outcome Group	No. of Patients
Group I	
Good recovery	34
Moderate disability	40
Total	74
Group II	
Severe disability	27
Vegetative	11
Total	38
Dead	77

that allowed them to be independent with minimal neurological deficit ("good recovery"). Twenty percent were severely disabled or vegetative.

The mortality rate in the HSC series is 41% (77/189), which more closely approximates the death rate reported in the adult series (Richmond: 34%; San Diego: 36%; Glasgow: 48%; The Netherlands and Los Angeles: 50% [11,19,20]). The HSC mortality is substantially greater than that recorded from some pediatric series (Bruce et al [6]: 6%; Ivan et al [21]: 24%; Pfenninger et al [10]: 21%; and Walker et al [9]: 12%). However, it does approximate the 32 to 38% mortality recently reported in other children's series [15,22,23].

Mortality Factors

The HSC mortality is a product of several factors, including initial GCS and the influence of multiple trauma on outcome, as well as referral patterns, initial triage, and air transport services to the hospital. It was also influenced by the phenomenon of craniovertebral disruption. This review has restricted the definition of "severe" brain injury to patients with a GCS of 7 or less and thus differs from those reports by Bruce et al [6] and Walker et al [9] where some patients were entered whose GCS was 8 or less at 6 hours. The inclusion of such patients may significantly enhance mortality and outcome. However, it is not to be assumed that a GCS of 8 or greater promises a normal outcome. In our review, 57 children admitted to the ICU were excluded because, based on their GCS values of 8 or greater, their brain injuries were not determined to be "severe" [12]. But only 35 of those children returned to normal.

Walker et al have stressed the impact of multiple trauma (defined as long bone fractures or ruptured abdominal organ) on outcome, noting that 80% of children with multiple injuries have associated brain trauma [9]. In their experience, 52% of all severely brain-injured children had associated severe multiple trauma, and the mortality was nearly twice as common in patients with severe brain injury and multiple trauma (32%) compared with children who had severe brain injury alone (17%). In the HSC review, 14 children died who had, in addition to a severe brain injury, major trauma to the chest, abdomen, or both; in all 14, hypovolemic shock was a problem. If these patients are excluded by virtue of their complex injury, then the mortality in this series from severe brain trauma diminishes to 36% (63/175).

We believe that initial triage and air transport services have an impact on the nature of the critically ill child reaching the hospital. Children who might have perished at the scene now arrive more expediently. Of the children in this review, 92% were admitted within 12 hours of trauma. We have deliberately excluded from this review children who died within 6 hours of trauma. But the efforts of ICU resuscitative techniques with multidiscipline participation are such that the period from 6 to 12 hours after trauma is of equal biological significance; it may be that patients who appeared viable at 6 hours may perish in the next 6 hours. If, on that basis, we exclude children in this series who died of brain injury within 12 hours of trauma or were declared brain dead by hour 12, then the overall mortality decreases to 34%.

Craniovertebral Disruption

It is moot testimony to roadside resuscitation and immediate triage that a few children in this series who died had arrived at our unit with very unstable vital signs relating to major craniovertebral disruption. Characteristically, traumatic lesions of the high cervical spine have been neatly categorized from the atlanto-occipital region caudal and as they involve articulating surfaces of adjacent structures or single bony units. Pang and Wilberger have studied the rare atlanto-occipital dislocation and note that the lesion may be more common than documented, because some patients do not survive long enough to be properly diagnosed [24]. Ten of the 14 patients they reviewed were less than 18 years of age, and 7 died shortly after admission to the hospital.

The occipital condyles and superior articular facets of the axis are related in a ball-in-socket motion, with "the atlas serving as an interposing ballbearing," [24]. Regrettably, the atlas has weak ligamentous attachments to the occiput and axis, hardly enough compensation in children who have small occipital condyles and shallow atlanto-articular surfaces [25]. Thus, forward slipping of the occiput on the atlas secondary to ligamentous rupture is more likely to occur in children than adults.

Direct brain stem injury from its distortion or from ischemia is the consequence of such dislocation, and the clinical features are related to the severity of the dislocation. In the milder forms, cardiorespiratory instability, nystagmus, decerebrate posturing, or flaccid extremity paralysis may be detected. Some of the brain-injured patients in the present review sustained cervico-medullary disconnection with respiratory arrest and were, for all intents and purposes, dead at the scene of trauma. However, resuscitative efforts there allowed them to be transported to our hospital.

In a companion report from our unit, 16 children suffered atlanto-occipital dislocation although the trauma was so devastating and the radiologic examinations were obtained under such precarious circumstances that the injuries were characterized by massive occipito-atlanto-axial commotion. The children ranged in age from 2 to 15 years; 7 were injured as motor vehicle passengers (5 died), 7 others were struck by vehicles (all died), and 2 were cyclists (both survived). All 12 children who died were observed to be pulseless and apneic right from the time of injury and required cardiopulmonary resuscitation at the scene. In all instances, autopsy confirmed high cervical cord and brain stem injury.

Given that there is a substantial mortality rate in children with severe primary brain injuries, many of whom seem destined to perish despite "sophisticated neurointensive care," [10] it may be inappropriate to consider mortality as the benchmark of outcome. As children's neurosurgeons, we have responsibilities as advocates for the prevention of the "primary injury," and as active therapists to halt the hypoxic, hypercarbic consequences of the "secondary injury" [9]. For those children who survive, we must be mindful that a "normal" neurological examination several months after trauma is not a measure of global outcome, as there may be significant deficits of intellectual development, memory, attention, perception, motor skills, and psychosocial adjustment that will require careful neuropsychological assessment and guidance.

REFERENCES

1. Hendrick EB, Harwood-Nash DC, Hudson AR. Head injuries in children: A survey of 4,465 consecutive cases at the Hospital for Sick Children, Toronto, Canada. Clin Neurosurg 1964;11:46–64.
2. Humphreys RP. Outcome of severe head injury in children. Concepts Pediatr Neurosurg 1983;3:191–201.
3. Marsh ML, Marshall LF, Shapiro HM. Neurosurgical intensive care. Ancsthesiology 1977;47:149–63.
4. Teasdale G, Jennett B. Assessment of coma and impaired consciousness. A practical scale. Lancet 1974;2:81–84.
5. Jennett B, Bond MR. Assessment of outcome after severe brain damage. Lancet 1975;1:480–84.
6. Bruce DA, Schut L, Bruno LA, Wood JH, Sutton LN. Outcome following severe head injuries in children. J Neurosurg 1978;48:679–88.
7. Bruce DA, Alavi A, Bilaniuk L, Dolinskas C, Obrist W, Uzzell B. Diffuse cerebral swelling following head injuries in children: The syndrome of "malignant brain edema." J Neurosurg 1981;54:170–78.
8. Amacher AL. Pediatric head injury: A national tragedy. Concepts Pediatr Neurosurg 1985;6:76–83.
9. Walker ML, Mayer TA, Storrs BB, Hylton PD. Pediatric head injury. Factors which influence outcome. Concepts Pediatr Neurosurg 1985;6:84–97.
10. Pfenninger J, Kaiser G, Lutschg J, Sutter M. Treatment and outcome of the severely head injured child. Intensive Care Med 1983;9:13–16.
11. Jennett B, Teasdale G. Management of head injuries. Contemp Neurol Ser. Vol. 20. Philadelphia: Davis, 1981.
12. Humphreys RP, Jaimovich R, Hendrick EB, Hoffman HJ. Severe head injuries in children. Concepts Pediatr Neurosurg 1983;4:230–42.
13. Langfitt TW. Measuring the outcome from head injuries. J Neurosurg 1978;48:673–78.
14. Becker DP, Miller JD, Ward JD, Greenberg RP, Young HF, Sakalas R. The outcome from severe head injury with early diagnosis and intensive management. J Neurosurg 1977;47:491–502.
15. Berger MS, Pitts LH, Lovely M, Edwards MSB, Bartkowski HM. Outcome from severe head injury in children and adolescents. J Neurosurg 1985;62:194–99.
16. Bruce DA, Raphaely RC, Goldberg AI, Zimmermann RA, Bilaniuk LT, Schut L, Kuhl DE. Pathophysiology, treatment and outcome following severe head injury in children. Childs Brain, 1979;5:174–91.

17. Langfitt TW, Gennarelli TA. Can the outcome from head injury be improved? J Neurosurg 1982;56:19–25.
18. Narayan RK, Greenberg RP, Miller JD, Enas GG, Choi SC, Kishore PRS, Selhorst JB, Lutz HA III, Becker DP. Improved confidence of outcome prediction in severe head injury. A comparative analysis of the clinical examination, multimodality evoked potentials, CT scanning and intracranial pressure. J Neurosurg 1981;54:751–62.
19. Bowers SA, Marshall LF. Outcome of 200 consecutive cases of severe head injury treated in San Diego County. A prospective analysis. Neurosurgery 1980;6:237–42.
20. Miller JD, Butterworth JF, Gudeman SK, Faulkner JE, Choi SC, Selhorst JB, Harbison JW, Lutz HA, Young HF, Becker DP. Further experience in the management of severe head injury. J Neurosurg 1981;54:289–99.
21. Ivan LP, Choo SH, Ventureyra ECG. Head injuries in childhood: A 2-year survey. Can Med Assoc J 1983;128:281–84.
22. Mahoney WJ, D'Souza BJ, Haller JA, Rogers MC, Epstein MH, Freeman JM. Long-term outcome of children with severe head trauma and prolonged coma. Pediatrics 1983;71:756–62.
23. Zuccarello M, Facco E, Zampieri P, Zarardi L, Andrioli GC. Severe head injury in children: Early prognosis and outcome. Childs Nerv Syst 1985;1:158–62.
24. Pang D, Wilberger JE Jr. Traumatic atlanto-occipital dislocation with survival: Case report and review. Neurosurgery 1980;7:503–8.
25. Wilberger JE Jr. Spinal cord injuries in children. Mount Kisco, NY. Futura Publishing Company, 1986:32–34.

Chapter 11

Gunshot Wounds to the Brain in Children

Michael E. Miner
Linda Ewing-Cobbs
Jack M. Fletcher
Dennis R. Kopaniky
Juan Cabrera
Paul Kaufmann

Children in the United States are more likely to die from a gunshot wound than from acquired immune deficiency syndrome (AIDS), brain tumors, heart disease, kidney disease, and a whole host of other well-known medical problems that have captured the attention of the public and the government. Children who are 15 years old or less cannot drive an automobile, are just starting high school, and generally have not had their first date but they account for nearly two thirds of all unintentional firearm deaths [1]. Not surprisingly there is a direct relationship between availability of firearms and firearm-related deaths [2]. However, even with the information currently available, this country has yet to develop a national policy that would restrict the availability of firearms among children.

The medical literature provides solid information relating to the issue of gun availability and mortality but minimal information on the results of intensive care for children with gunshot wounds to the brain. This is in sharp contrast to the information available in adult patients with gunshot wounds. We have been in a unique position to evaluate children with gunshot wounds to the brain very early after injury and to use an aggressive treatment regimen. This then prompted us to attempt to mobilize community resources to affect the problem.

MATERIALS AND METHODS

Ninety-five children less than 16 years of age were treated for gunshot wounds at University Children's Hospital at Hermann (UCHH) during calendar years 1981 through 1986. Thirty-three (35%) were shot in the brain. This represents 21% of the number of adults shot in the brain who were seen at our institution during the same period. Data from their records were recorded prospectively on standardized forms. Each of the 33 children with gunshot wounds to the brain was flown to UCHH by helicopter ambulance and arrived within two hours after injury. Before helicopter transport, each patient's wounds were bandaged, a large-bore intravenous (IV) tube was inserted, and an initial dose of anticonvulsants and antibiotics was administered. Intravenous mannitol (0.5 g/kg) and endotracheal intubation were instituted in each child who could not follow commands.

In the emergency center a neurologic examination was coded in terms of the Glasgow Coma Score and a thorough physical examination and laboratory evaluation were promptly performed. Brain CT scans were obtained immediately on patients who were not in shock. Patients were subsequently taken directly to the operating room for debridement of their wound. The only exceptions were those patients who were hemodynamically unstable or who were neurologically devastated (Glasgow Coma Score = 3, pupils dilated and not reactive to light, absent occulocephalic reflexes). All of these patients either died in the emergency center or were taken to the intensive care unit (ICU) for further resuscitation before being committed to surgery.

Intracranial pressure (ICP) was monitored as part of the surgical procedure in all patients except those who could follow commands before surgery, and had a normal cranial nerve examination, and had CT evidence of visible pontine cisterns, and a midline shift of less than 4 mm. The basic surgical procedure was the removal of all devitalized brain tissue and accessible foreign bodies. Antibiotics were continued for 7 days. Anticonvulsants were started in the emergency room and continued for a minimum of six months. All patients were initially treated in the pediatric critical care unit. Elevated ICP was defined as greater than 20 mm Hg and was managed by a standardized regimen that included a hierarchy of sedation, muscle relaxants, hyperventilation, osmotic diuretics, and barbiturate coma. All surviving patients had a follow-up CT brain scan between days 3 and 5 postinjury. Further contrast-enhanced CT brain scans were obtained weekly for one month if the child remained in the hospital. At six months another brain image was obtained (either CT or magnetic resonance image).

Survivors were evaluated at 6 and 12 months postinjury by the Glasgow Outcome Scale, which has the following categories: (1) dead; (2) vegetative; (3) severe disability (not able to function independently and requiring substantial home care or institutionalization as a result of intellectual or physical impairment); (4) moderate disability (able to function independently at a reduced level because of personality, intellectual, or physical differences compared with preinjury status); and (5) good (resumption of preinjury activities with minimal neurologic deficit or apparent change in personality or school performance) [3].

RESULTS

Of the 33 children shot in the brain, 23 were boys and 10 were girls. Age at injury ranged from 8 months to 15 years. Nineteen died and 14 survived; the gross mortality rate was 58%. Figure 11.1 shows when these deaths occurred and when the survivors were discharged from the hospital. Fourteen died, or 74% of all deaths occurred, within 24 hours of injury. Of the survivors, 2 had good recoveries, 9 were moderately disabled, and 3 had severe disabilities at 6 months after injury. No patients were left in a vegetative state.

Although 70% of these children were boys, the mortality rate for the boys was 48% and that for the girls was 80%. This difference was primarily a reflection of there being more older girls successful at suicide. Although older children had a higher mortality rate (see Figure 11.2), among those accidentally injured, the mortality rate was no different in any age group, nor was there a difference in mortality between girls and boys.

Glasgow Coma Score and Outcome

As seen in Table 11.1, only 5 of these 33 children presented with Glasgow Coma Scores greater than 8, but all 5 made adequate recoveries (Glasgow outcomes of good recovery or moderate disability). Seven patients had initial Glasgow Coma Scores of 6 to 8. Of these children, 1 died, 2 were severely

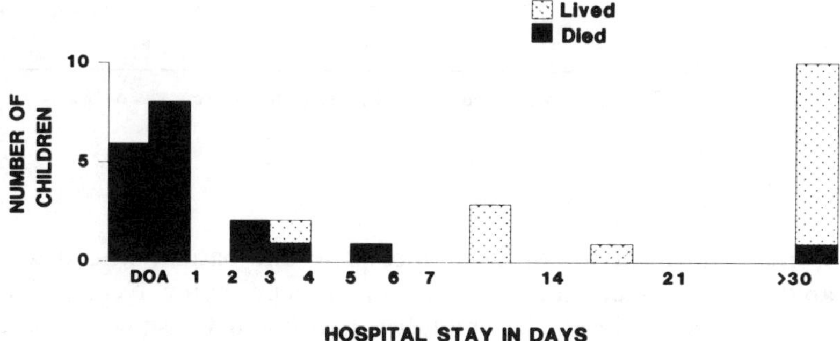

Figure 11.1   The overwhelming majority of patients who died did so within the first 24 hours after injury. However, nearly two thirds of the survivors were hospitalized for more than one month. This information suggests that there truly is a group of children with lethal injuries after gunshot wounds to the brain.

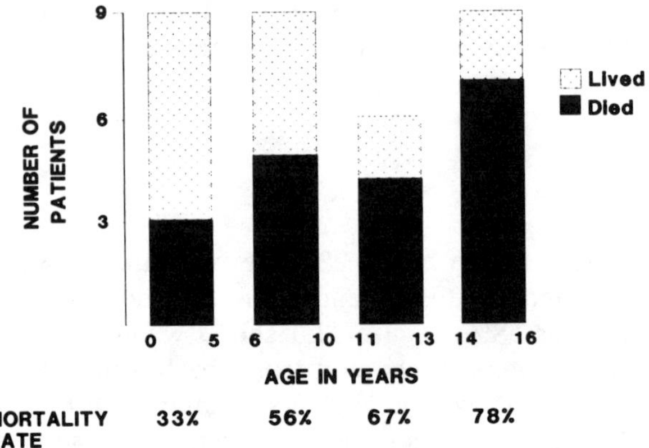

Figure 11.2   Age-related mortality in children with gunshot wounds to the brain. Mortality increased progressively with age. In older children this was primarily influenced by suicide attempts; these occurred only in children over the age of 10 years and were lethal in 80% of the cases.

Table 11.1   Outcome in Children Six Months Postinjury Compared with Glasgow Coma Score (GCS) on Hospital Admission[a]

Initial GCS	No. of Patients with Glasgow Outcome of:					Total Patients	%
	1	*2*	*3*	*4*	*5*		
9–15				3	2	5	15
6–8	1	0	2	4	0	7	21
3–5	18	0	1	2	0	21	64
Total	19	0	3	9	2	33	100

[a]Overall morality rate for gunshot wounds to the brain in children was 57%.

disabled, and 4 have moderate disabilities. The one patient who died in this group rapidly deteriorated and died in the emergency center. Nearly two-thirds of children shot in the brain (21 children), had initial Glasgow Coma Scores of 3 to 5; 18 of them (86%) died. Two made adequate recoveries, and one was severely disabled. The obvious relationship between an initial Glasgow Coma Score of 3 to 5 and survival was supported by a chi-square test (with one degree of freedom = 18.7, P < 0.001).

Trajectory and Survival

The entrance wound was on the right side in 21 of these children and on the left in 12. All 11 of those who attempted suicide were right handed and had right-sided entrance wounds. Thus, in those not attempting suicide, the entrance wound was on the right in 10 and on the left in 12. The overall mortality in patients with right-sided entrance wounds was 67%; for left-sided entrance wounds it was 42%. However, this difference was not present in patients with accidental gunshot wounds to the brain.

The path of the wound was critical to survival. Only two of the patients had a single lobe of the brain injured, and they both survived with good outcomes. Eleven had trajectories through multiple lobes of the same hemisphere, and three of these patients died. Twenty of the children had trajectories through both hemispheres, and 16 died (80%). As seen in Table 11.2, the correlation between bihemispheric injuries and death was highly significant (chi square with 1 degree of freedom $= 10.6$, $P < 0.005$). Only three children had through and through injuries, and one survived.

Although the trajectory of the bullet significantly influenced mortality, the caliber of the bullet did not. The type of gun used was relatively unimportant compared with how close it was to the head and which direction it was pointing when fired.

Circumstance of Shooting

The cause of these shootings varied with age. Eleven children attempted suicide; 9 died. All were 10 years of age or older, and they accounted for more than half of the 21 children over age 10 years. Thirteen other children had either inflicted gunshot wounds on themselves while playing with a pistol or been shot by a peer who was playing with a gun. All but 2 of these children were 10 years old or less. All five who died while playing with guns were 10 years old or less. Two boys were shot when a gun was used to settle an argument between siblings; one died. Three children were shot while they were

Table 11.2   Chi-Square Analysis of Bullet Trajectory Injuries in Children

	No. of Patients Who:		
Bullet Trajectory	*Lived*	*Died*	*Total*
Bihemispheric	4	16	20
One hemisphere	10	3	13
Total	14	19	33

onlookers to criminal acts. Only one child was shot during a criminal act. The father shot his 15-year-old son as the boy was beating his mother. Although no criminal charges were filed against the father, that child was the only one even suspected of being involved in a criminal act. One child survived a gunshot wound resulting from a hunting accident. The circumstances surrounding the shooting of two children who were dead on arrival at the emergency center were never ascertained. There was a significant relationship between mortality and suicide attempt as compared with the mortality from all other modalities (chi square with one degree of freedom = 4.2, $P < 0.05$).

Increased ICP

ICP was monitored in 18 patients. Six did not have ICP monitoring because they died in the emergency room due to hemodynamic instability complicated by coagulation defects. The outcome for five other patients was considered hopeless because of their neurologic deficit (Glasgow Coma Score = 3, bilaterally fixed dilated pupils, and bihemispheric bullet trajectory), and they died within 24 hours of injury. Another 4 patients were not thought to need ICP monitoring because of their good clinical status.

Of the 18 patients whose ICP was monitored, 9 died. Eight died who had ICP values greater than 40 mm Hg, and one died of pneumonia a month after his injury although his ICP had been controllable below 30 mm Hg. He had been in a persistent vegetative state from the time of his injury until his death. Of the survivors, three did not have any ICP measurement greater than 20 mm Hg and required minimal treatment. Two others had ICP values that were greater than 20 mm Hg but, with treatment (muscle relaxants, analgesics, mannitol, and hyperventilation), did not exceed 30 mm Hg. Four patients had ICP values greater than 40 mm Hg in spite of the same medical and surgical management. Two were treated in barbiturate coma. Of these four, two had a severe disability at 6 months and two were moderately disabled. Thus, of the three patients with severe disabilities at 6 months, two had had high ICP values and one was not monitored for ICP because of an enormous shotgun blast that removed most of his left parietal, temporal, and frontal lobe although he was able to follow commands when admitted to the hospital. All patients with normal ICP had good or moderate disabilities at 6 months after injury.

Weapon

Twenty-seven of these 33 children (82%) were shot with pistols. Four were shot with rifles, and two were shot with shotguns. The caliber of the weapon alone did not predict survival or morbidity. However, all those shot with a rifle died.

Table 11.3 Neurologic Deficits in 14 Children Six
Months Postinjury

Deficit	*No. of Patients*
None	1
Hemiparesis	10
Blind in one eye	1
Blind in both eyes	1
Deaf in one ear	1
Attentional/memory deficits	13
Speech/language deficits	5

Survivors: Complications and Disabilities

In one child a sterile brain abscess developed that was evacuated a month after
his injury. Seizures occurred in two children at 7 and 11 months after injury.
In both cases the seizures were readily controlled with phenytoin.

We evaluated outcome 6 months after injury in the 14 survivors. Two
had a good recovery at 6 months, 9 had moderate disabilities, and 3 were
severely disabled. One child had no detectable abnormalities six months after
her injury. However, 10 had signs of a hemiparesis, 2 were blind in one or
both eyes, 1 was deaf in one ear, 13 had attentional or memory deficits, and
5 had language deficits requiring treatment. At six months after injury nearly
80% had an adequate neurologic recovery as judged by the Glasgow Outcome
Scale (Table 11.3), but many deficits remained. At one year, one child had
improved from severely disabled to moderately disabled and another child had
improved from moderately disabled to a good outcome.

DISCUSSION

Experience with gunshot wounds to the brain in adults would suggest that
survival can be accurately predicted from the bullet's trajectory and the patient's
initial neurological status [4]. This has prompted many clinicians to assume a
rather dismal prognosis in patients with severe brain injury following gunshot
wounds [5–9]. Kaufman et al identified two patients with severe brain injury
caused by gunshot wounds who made impressive recoveries and has argued
that a more aggressive approach should be taken to patients with these injuries
[10]. However, except perhaps for more rapid triage, the management of the
adult with a gunshot wound to the brain appears little changed over the past
several years. Indeed, experience and the literature available on civilian gunshot
wounds do not support the making of more effort in the moribund adult

following gunshot wounds [5–9]. On the other hand, similar data are not available in children. Reports that children fare better than adults after severe brain injuries would encourage an aggressive approach to gunshot-wounded children [11–13]. Therefore, because we have been in a position of evaluating patients quite early after injury, we wanted to test the notion that early aggressive surgery and a standard treatment protocol resulted in a high salvage rate for children severely brain injured due to gunshot wounds.

Despite routine evaluation of children within two hours after injury and an aggressive treatment regimen, one third either died of hemodynamic instability or were so neurologically devastated that prudence contraindicated surgical treatment. A total of 74% of the deaths occurred within the first 24 hours after injury, suggesting that those patients had a lethal injury from the onset. This may simply reflect on Cushing's observations at the end of World War I that the earlier one evaluates severely injured patients the higher the number of untreatable injuries [14]. There may be a lower limit of salvageability for severely injured children with gunshot wounds to the brain [15].

No series are available that specifically detail the outcome of children with gunshot wounds to the brain. Compared with data published from two other large urban populations it does appear that we in Houston, Texas, are treating a particularly great number of children with gunshot wounds, and that these wounds are more frequently to the brain [16,17]. This may simply be a reflection of local referral practice, but it may also reflect a relatively permissive attitude toward gun safety. It must also be noted that there is a significant literature indicating that air rifle injuries may also result in severe, permanent neurologic injuries in children [18,19].

Fifty-eight percent of the 34 children died, which is comparable to adult mortality rates for similar injuries [5–9]. In keeping with observations in adult patients, neither the victim's age or gender, nor the caliber of the bullet, were predictors of survival in children shot in the brain. However, a poor initial neurologic evaluation, high ICP, bihemispheric bullet trajectory, and the intent to commit suicide were robust predictors of mortality [4]. A poor initial neurologic exam, defined as no response or only decerebrate or decorticate responses to painful stimuli, strikingly identified whether the wound was mortal. However, two children who initially had only decerebrate posturing to painful stimuli were left with moderate disabilities. Therefore, in the child, decerebrate or decorticate posturing after gunshot wounds to the brain is not a contraindication to aggressive treatment. ICP values greater than 40 mm Hg correlated with a mortal injury in two-thirds of the patients, and half of the patients who survived such high ICP were severely disabled. In those patients who had a more normal ICP, however, there were no mortalities and the outcomes were acceptable. Bullet trajectory was strongly linked to survival. Children wishing to commit suicide shot themselves through both hemispheres, and such injuries had a mortality rate in excess of 80%. This 80% figure held up in other cases in which the trajectory of the bullet was across both hemispheres. Thus, the high mortality rate associated with the intent to commit suicide was linked to the trajectory of the bullet, but bihemispheric injuries did not necessarily predict that the child had attempted suicide.

The morbidity from the wounds in these children may be considered somewhat less than that observed in adults, in that none of these children was left in a persistent vegetative state [5–9]. However, even one year after injury the daily lives of the survivors were affected in all but one child, to say nothing of the effect on the families and friends of all of the patients. All of the children left with moderate disabilities had deficits that affected their ability to learn even one year after their injuries. Two thirds of the survivors had a hemiparesis, and one-third had language disorders still requiring treatment. The children with severe deficits are particularly worrisome. Although they are in school, their performance is considerably below that of their peer group. We are greatly concerned that their future may hold a poor outcome with regard to educability and employment. In addition, further medical care to date has included second operations for 50% of the survivors (usually cranioplasty). The potential for the further development of major medical effects such as seizures also remains quite high. Thus, we are encouraged by the results at one year but remain very concerned about the long-term effects of these injuries.

Perhaps the most striking observations in these children were the circumstances surrounding their injuries. One-third were attempting suicide. This sobering fact is even more poignant in that all of the suicide attempts were performed with a loaded handgun that was unsecured in the home. No child stole a gun, and only one loaded it himself. Firearms are the most common way that young people commit suicide, and it appears that suicide is on the rise in the United States [20]. All of the children that we evaluated were less than 16 years old. The youngest child who committed suicide with a gunshot wound to the brain was in the fourth grade.

Forty percent of these children were playing with a handgun when they were shot. None of these children were stealing or crazed by drugs, and only one was involved in a crime of violence. Overall, 80% were shot with a handgun. Even though the "appropriate" use of firearms is difficult to define regarding a child, only one child was involved in a hunting accident. This is in concert with the data from Patterson and Smith. They surveyed 150 families who attended the pediatric clinic at the University of Texas Medical Branch, Galveston [21]. Over one third of the families had at least one gun in their home, and over half noted that the gun was always loaded and ready to use.

Our experience would indicate that virtually all of these children's injuries could have been prevented if handguns were less readily accessible. Unfortunately, handguns primarily made of plastic may soon be available at low costs. These weapons have been promoted as "dishwasher safe" and "particularly attractive for women" [1]. Such weapons will undoubtedly be found by children. Clearly, increasing the accessibility of handguns is detrimental to children.

HOUSTON CHILD-SAFE COMMITTEE

During the first two months of 1986, 13 children were shot with a gun. Eleven were shot in the brain, and six of these children died. All were cases of children shooting children. None of the children were involved in criminal actions, nor was their consciousness clouded by drugs. Most of the shootings occurred in the home, but two occurred on school grounds. This was such an increase in the usual rate of injury that it appeared to fulfill the criteria of an epidemic. A group of local citizens came together who represented a diverse range of interests. Members of the National Rifle Association, the Chief of the Houston Police Department, the Superintendent of the Houston Independent School System, physicians, nurses, and interested parents attempted to bring together the vast resources of the community. The goal of the Houston Child-Safe Committee was merely to inform the citizenry that making guns unavailable to small children could save lives. We particularly stressed that a loaded handgun in the home was much more likely to kill a friend or loved one than a villain [22]. A secondary goal was to make individuals aware that if they had a gun in the home, they must be responsible for it. That meant that they were to exercise appropriate safety precautions. The goals were generally accepted but the methods to accomplish them were not agreed on by all.

However, within six weeks a 30-minute film was made and scheduled for prime time viewing on one of the local television stations, newspaper articles were published both in the news and editorial sections, bumper stickers were distributed, grocery bags were imprinted with safety slogans, the concerns were discussed during religious worship services, and billboards were put up throughout the city (see Figure 11.3). There were proclamations from the mayor, and an enormous number of children were reached by the police department's educational division. Many people representing many areas of Houston, the fourth largest city in the United States, tried to affect a health problem without calling for government regulation.

The benefits were great. Most important, the death rate from accidental gunshot wounds to the brain has decreased greatly. For the twelve months after the initiation of this educational effort, no child under the age of 16 years was killed in Houston, Texas. However, it was also beneficial to see that even a large community could quickly mobilize its resources to change a problem. But a very real question is: Will the effect last? Unfortunately, the answer is probably no [23]. However, as with many preventive campaigns, it may make it easier for the next effort to be effective because the groundwork has been laid and need not be repeated. Such efforts can be rewarding, but there is also a place for responsible legislation. It is difficult to believe that a law mandating a waiting period before the purchase of a handgun is detrimental. Requiring the buyer to demonstrate competency and a knowledge of fundamental safety precautions is no more of an infringement on his or her independence than a driver's license examination. Furthermore, it should be apparent that in our

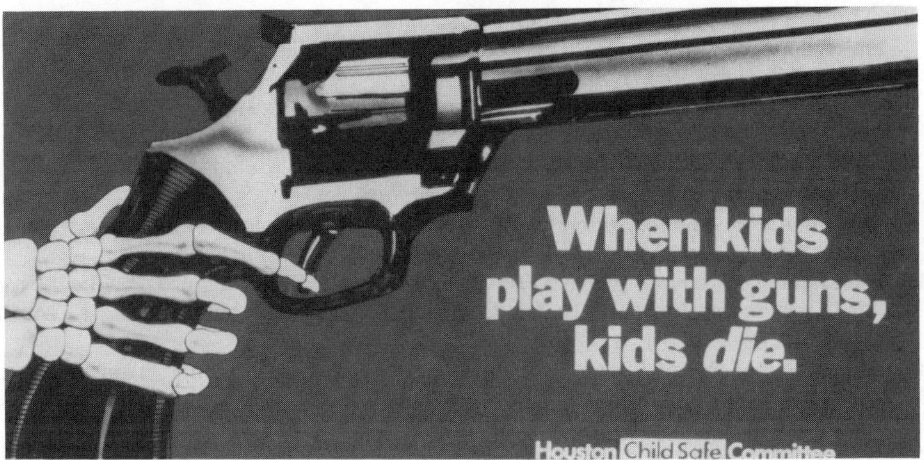

Figure 11.3 Billboard, appearing in more than 75 locations in the greater Houston area, that was used to heighten awareness of gunshot wounds in children.

litiginous climate the question of negligent homicide is going to be raised and a deep pocket identified. Therefore, it seems in the best interest of both gun advocates and antagonists to develop a rational approach to gun safety that is not currently in practice. Certainly, it would reduce a major cause of death and disability in children.

ACKNOWLEDGMENT

This work was supported in part by NIH Grant NS21889: Neurobehaviorial Outcome of Head Injury in Children.

REFERENCES

1. Wintemute GJ, Teret SP, Kraus JF, Wright MA, Bradfield G. When children shoot children. JAMA 1987;258:3107–9.
2. Teret SP, Wintemute GJ. Handgun injuries: The epidemologic evidence for assessing legal responsibility. Hamline Law Rev 1983;6:341–50.
3. Jennett B, Bond M. Assessment of outcome after severe brain damage: A practical scale. Lancet 1975;1:480–4.
4. Nagib MG, Rockswold GL, Sherman RS, Lagaard MW. Civilian gunshot wounds to the brain: Prognosis and management. Neurosurgery 1986;18:533–37.
5. Hernsniemi J. Penetrating craniocerebral wounds in civilians. Acta Neurochir 1979;49:199–205.

6. Hubschman O, Shapiro K, Baden M, Shulman K. Craniocerebral gunshot injuries in civilian practice: Prognostic criteria and surgical managment experience with 82 cases. J Trauma 1979;19:6–12.

7. Lillard PL. Five year experience with penetrating craniocerebral gunshot wounds. Surg Neurol 1978;9:79–83.

8. Raimondi AJ, Samuelson GH. Craniocerebral gunshot wounds in civilian practice. J Neurosurg 1970;32:647–53.

9. Sherman WP, Apuzzo MCJ, Heiden JS, Peterson VT, Weiss MH. Gunshot wounds to the brain: A civilian experience. West J Med 1980;132:99–105.

10. Kaufman HH, Loyola WP, Makela ME, Frankowski RF, Wagner DP, Gildenberg PL. Civilian gunshot wounds: The limits of salvageability. Acta Neurochir (Wien) 1983;67:115–25.

11. Alberico AM, Ward JD, Choi SC, Marmarou A, Young HF. Outcome after severe head injury: Relationship to mass lesions, diffuse injury, and ICP course in pediatric and adult patients. J Neurosurg 1987;67:648–56.

12. Berger MS, Pitts LH, Lovely M, Edwards MSB, Bartkowski HM. Outcome from severe head injury in children and adolescents. J Neurosurg 1985;62:194–99.

13. Bruce DA, Schut L, Bruno LA, Wood JH, Sutton LN. Outcome following severe head injuries in children. J Neurosurg 1978;48:679–88.

14. Cushing H. Notes on penetrating wounds of the brain. Br Med J 1918;1:221–26.

15. Clifton GL, Grossman RG, Makela ME, Miner ME, Handel S, Sadhu V. Neurological course and correlated computerized tomography findings after severe closed head injury. J Neurosurg 1980;52:611–24.

16. Valentine J, Blocker S, Chang J. Gunshot injuries in children. J Trauma 1984;24:952–56.

17. Barlow B, Niemirska M, Gandhi RP. Ten years' experience with pediatric gunshot wounds. J Pediat Surg 1982;17:927–32.

18. Blocker S, Cohn D, Chang JHT. Serious air rifle injuries in children. Pediatrics 1982;69:751–54.

19. Miner ME, Cabrera JA, Ford E, Ewing-Cobbs L, Amling J. Intracranial penetration due to BB air rifle injuries. Neurosurgery 1986;19:952–54.

20. Bolt JH, Moscicki EK. Firearms and youth suicide. Am J Public Health 1986;76:1240–42.

21. Patterson PJ, Smith LR. Firearms in the home and child safety. Am J Dis Child 1987;141:221–23.

22. Kellermann AL, Reay DT. Protection or peril? An analysis of firearm-related deaths in the home. N Eng J Med 1986;314:1557–60.

23. Heins M, Kahn R, Bjordnal J. Gunshot wounds in children. Am J Public Health 1974;64:326–30.

Chapter 12

Applications of Multimodality Sensory Evoked Responses in the Pediatric Intensive Care Unit

James W. Hall III
Denise A. Tucker
Stephen A. Fletcher
Rolf Habersang

Multimodality (auditory, somatosensory, and visual) evoked responses (SERs) can be recorded in intensive care unit (ICU) settings to evaluate the neurologic status of critically ill patients [1–4]. For the most part, existing reports describe the use of SERs in adult populations. There are fewer investigations of the possible roles of SERs in the management of children with acute brain injury [4–9].

At our institutions, audiology personnel are routinely involved in SER monitoring of the central nervous system (CNS) in pediatric ICU patients. As indicated in Table 12.1, we have applied one or more modalities of SERs in the evaluation of more than 250 children with acute brain pathologies. We have particular experience in the application of auditory evoked responses in traumatic brain injury in children.

METHODS

Age of the subject population ranged from 1 week to 15 years. Physiologic parameters for the population are summarized in Table 12.2. Although average values were within acceptable limits, the group was heterogeneous. There were, for example, patients whose status was characterized by hypothermia, hypotension, increased intracranial pressure (ICP), and hypoxia.

Table 12.1 Summary of Authors' Clinical Experience with Sensory Evoked Response Measurement of 237 Children in the Pediatric Intensive Care Unit

	Patients	
Clinical Entity	*(n)*	*(%)*
Traumatic brain injury	102	43
Meningitis	62	26
Hypoxic/ischemic insult	23	10
Seizures	18	8
Hydrocephalus	15	6
Other	17	7

Table 12.2 Summary of Physiologic Variables at the Time of Auditory Brain Stem Response Assessment for 102 Children with Acute Brain Injury[a]

Variable[b]	*Mean*	*SD*	*Range*
Temperature	37	± 1	30–40
Mean arterial pressure	86	± 17	49–102
Intracranial pressure	20	± 18	0–109
Cerebral perfusion pressure	67	± 27	−12–124
PaO_2	117	± 40	22–203
$PaCO_2$	29	± 16	10–42

[a]There were 190 test sessions.
[b]Temperature is given in degrees celsius; all other values represent millimeters of mercury.

All patients underwent SER measurement at bedside with commercially available equipment (Nicolet CA-1000). Initial SER testing was carried out within 48 hours of hospital admission in 70% of the series. Most patients underwent serial measurement during the acute phase after injury. The test protocol in the present study was recently described elsewhere [4]. Briefly, stimuli used to elicit the evoked responses for the three modalities were as follows:

1. Auditory brain stem response (ABR). Acoustic clicks, 0.1 msec in duration, were presented monaurally to the right and left ears at a rate of 21.1/sec and an intensity of 85 dB hearing level (Re: adult click behavioral threshold) via TDH-39 earphones. Two replicable ABR waveforms were averaged for 2,000 repetitions of the stimulus.

2. Somatosensory evoked response (SSER). Electrical pulses, 0.1 msec in duration, were delivered to the right and left median nerves at the wrist via a bipolar surface electrode array at a rate of 5.1/sec and an intensity sufficient to generate a distinct thumb twitch (generally 5 to 15 mamp). Two replicable SSER waveforms were averaged for 500 repetitions of the stimulus.
3. Visual evoked response (VER). Flash photic stimuli of undetermined duration were presented monocularly to the right and left eyes (eyelids closed) at a rate of 2.8/sec and an intensity easily detected by the tester, under identical presentation conditions, through goggles. Two replicable VER waveforms were averaged for 500 repetitions of the stimulus.

Evoked responses were detected with surface electroencephalogram (EEG) electrodes placed on the scalp. For ABR measurement, electrodes were located at a midline, high forehead site (voltage positive) and earlobe or mastoid ipsilateral to the stimulus (voltage negative) with a common ground on the low forehead (nasion). The SSER was measured simultaneously with two channels. Recording electrodes for channel 1 were located at Erb's point (the depression just above the clavicle superficial to the brachial plexus) on the stimulated side (voltage negative) and the forehead (voltage positive) with a plate electrode for ground on the forearm approximately 15 mm proximal to the stimulating electrodes. For the second channel, recording electrodes were located over the parietal cortex contralateral to the stimulus (voltage negative) and the forehead (voltage positive) with the common forearm ground. The VER was also recorded with two channels. The negative electrode was located over the right occipital region (the 02 site, according to the 10-20 EEG system) for the first channel and over the left occipital region (01) for the second channel. The two channels shared a positive electrode site (forehead) and ground site (vertex).

RESULTS

Findings for SSERs and VERs are illustrated by case reports. Correlations among group data for these SERs were difficult to interpret due to considerable variability among subjects in factors known to influence the response. These included, in particular, age, among subjects 8 years and younger; physical dimensions, for the somatosensory modality; and consistency of the flash photic stimuli, for the visual modality. SSERs were the most effective modality of the evoked responses for monitoring cerebral integrity and lateralizing the site of cerebral lesion in traumatic brain injury. VERs had relatively greater sensitivity to cerebral dysfunction associated with hydrocephalus but did not typically add appreciably to information provided by evoked responses in the auditory and somatosensory modalities for other clinical entities. These points will be highlighted with case reports to follow.

The ABR offered the most reliable index of brain stem function in the comatose child. Initial ABR findings were within normal limits for more than

75% of the group. Therefore, the ABR could be used to document subsequent deterioration of brain stem status in those patients in whom secondary CNS pathophysiology developed. The ABR was also extremely valuable in assessing peripheral auditory status in patients at risk for hearing impairment, for example, patients with meningitis or traumatic brain injury [10,11].

Correlations among ABR interwave latencies and clinical findings are displayed in Table 12.3. Data are reported only for patients with a body temperature of 36 to 38°C at ABR testing, because deviations in body temperature have documented effects on response latency. There was a strong association among brain stem transmission time, as measured by ABR, and established clinical findings, including mean arterial pressure (MAP), intracranial pressure (ICP), and calculated perfusion pressure (CPP), as well as the pupillary response to light. As will be demonstrated in case reports to follow, however, relationships among ABR and these physiologic parameters are not invariable. ABR findings and arterial oxygen tension (PaO_2) were not highly correlated. The significance of the relationship between ABR and blood gases is difficult to assess; unlike the other physiologic values, blood gas data were collected not at the time of SER evaluation but at some point less than four hours before testing.

CASE REPORTS

Case 1: ABR Versus VER and SER

The patient, a 2-month-old girl, had been riding in an unsecured car seat during a motor vehicle accident. Emergency CT scanning upon hospital admission revealed left hemisphere edema, greatest in the temporal lobe region. In the pediatric ICU she received standard medical therapy for increased ICP.

Table 12.3 Correlation among Physiologic Parameters and Auditory Brain Stem Response (ABR) Latencies for 102 Normothermic Brain-Injured Children (129 Test Sessions)[a]

	ABR Component Latency		
Physiologic Variable	*I–III*	*III–V*	*I–V*
Mean arterial pressure	+	−	−
Intracranial pressure	+ +	+ +	+ +
Cerebral perfusion pressure	+ +	+ +	+ +
PaO_2	+	−	+
$PaCO_2$	−	−	−
Pupillary response	+ +	+ +	+ +

[a]Symbols: + +, $P < 0.01$; +, $P < 0.05$; −, not significant at $P = 0.05$.

Initial SERs were carried out within 12 hours postadmission. At the time of testing, vital signs were normal. Neurologic examination showed pupils equal and reactive to light. ICP, as monitored at the fontanel, was 6 mm Hg. An ABR was reliably recorded bilaterally. Brain stem transmission times (wave I–V latency interval) were within age-matched normal limits (see top waveform in Figure 12.1). At the same test session, as illustrated in Figure 12.2, there were no apparent cortical components for the VER and SSER. A peripheral component was observed for each sensory modality.

At this time, because of the markedly abnormal VER and SSER findings, the attending physician removed and recalibrated the ICP monitor. Upon replacement of the monitor, an ICP of 109 mm Hg was recorded. The child was treated aggressively for increased ICP. Repeat SER recordings were made daily.

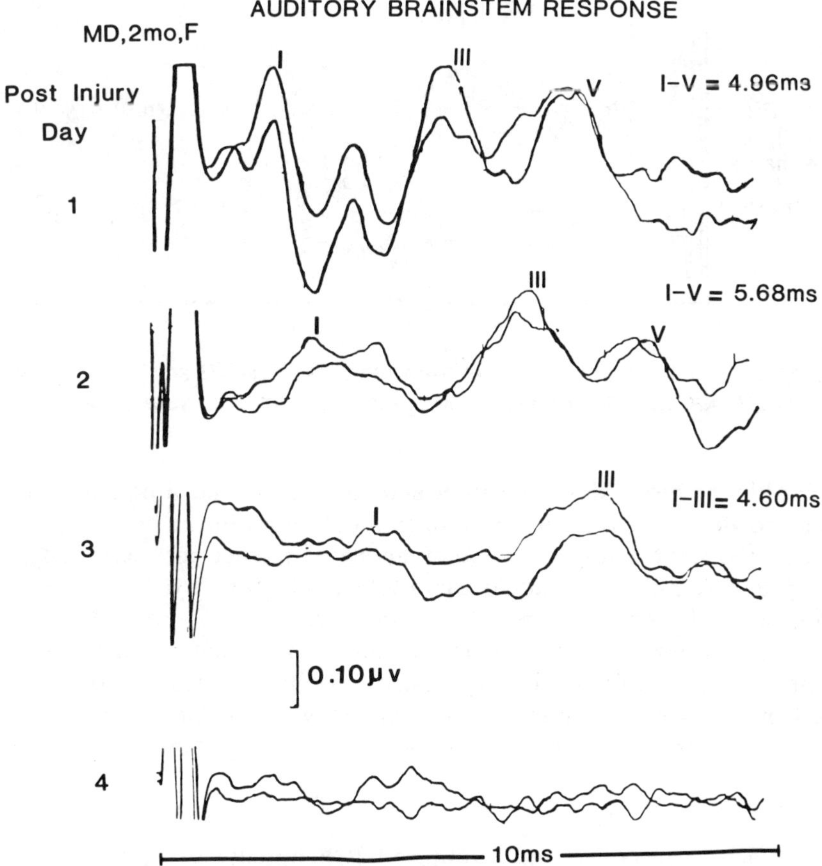

Figure 12.1   Serial auditory brain stem response (ABR) recordings for a two-month-old girl with a closed head injury (case 1).

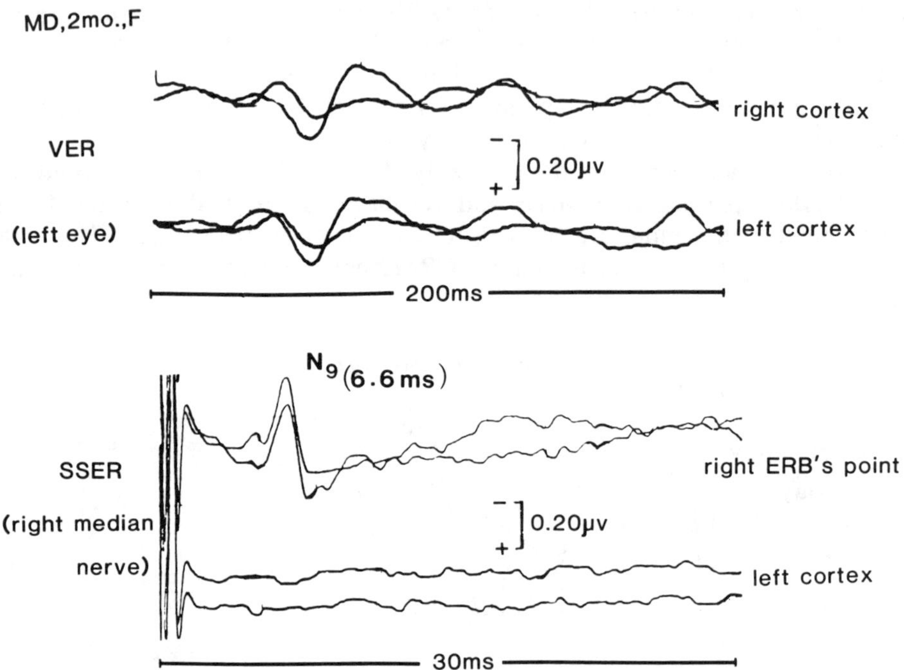

Figure 12.2   Initial somatosensory evoked response (SSER) and visual evoked response (VER) waveforms for case 1. No cortical components were observed.

Within the next 3 days, the VER and SSER cortical components remained absent and the ABR reflected progressive deterioration of brain stem status. Although the wave I (eighth nerve component) latency increased, suggesting evolving peripheral (e.g., middle ear) otologic abnormality, brain stem transmission times also became significantly prolonged (see Figure 12.1). Repeated CT showed extensive edema, which included white matter, in the posterior fossa and into the midbrain. By day 4 postinjury, there was no evoked response for any modality at maximum stimulus intensity levels. EEG was absent (not shown). Life support systems were removed, and the patient died.

Comment

ABR, pupillary response and monitored ICP initially suggested brain stem integrity and argued against impending neurologic decompensation. Absence of the SSER and VER cortical components, in contrast, was evidence of serious cortical pathology, perhaps associated with cerebral edema noted on the emergency CT, and therefore cast doubt on the validity of monitored ICP. Subsequent serial ABRs documented progressive deterioration of brain stem CNS status, presumably secondary to ischemia [12–16], and ultimately provided neurophysiologic correlation of CT evidence of midbrain compression. Finally, multimodality SERs served as ancillary indexes of brain death.

Case 2. Multimodality SERs in Outcome

The patient was a 12-year-old boy who sustained an accidental gunshot wound while hunting. Upon arrival at the emergency center, he was comatose. CT revealed a bullet track through the left frontal, temporal, and occipital lobes. A fracture in the left occipital region and bone fragments in the left occiput were also noted. The child underwent craniotomy with decompression and then was transferred to the pediatric ICU. Medical protocol for elevated ICP was begun.

ABR measurement was made immediately after surgery. Normal waveforms were recorded bilaterally (Figure 12.3). Brain stem transmission times

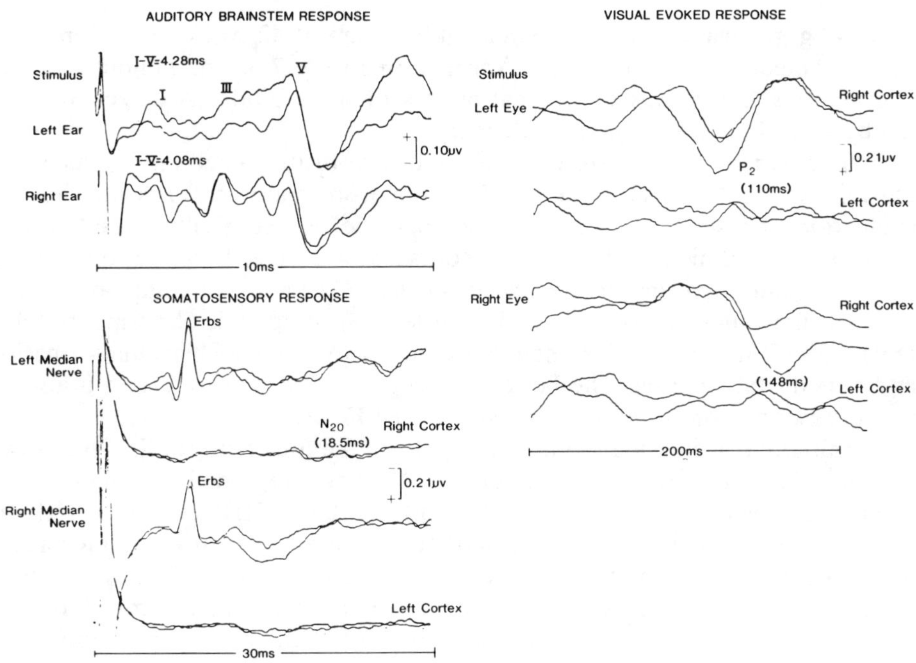

Figure 12.3　Auditory, somatosensory, and visual evoked response waveforms for a 12-year-old boy with a gunshot wound to the head and left cerebral hemisphere damage (case 2).

(wave I–V latency interval) were within normal limits. When a pressure bandage was removed the following day, initial SSER and VER assessments were completed (see Figure 12.3). A clear and reliable VER was recorded over the right occipital region, but there was no apparent response on the left. Median nerve somatosensory stimulation produced a parietal component of very small amplitude on the right and no cortical response on the left. In combination, then, the ABR indicated brain stem integrity, whereas SSER and VER results provided evidence of left hemisphere cerebral dysfunction, consistent with the lesion seen with CT scanning.

The patient's status improved, and he was later transferred to a rehabilitation center for speech, physical, and occupational therapy. During the course of rehabilitation, his verbal expression developed from telegraphic speech to speech characterized by word-finding problems and circumlocutions. Sentences were incomplete and reduced in length. Reading and writing abilities were severely limited. Acute SSER and VER abnormalities on the left served as a prognostic indicator of long-term speech and language outcome.

Case 3. ABR in Hydrocephalus

A 3,147-g girl was born to a 25-year-old woman at 42 weeks gestational age by spontaneous vaginal delivery. Apgar scores were 7 at one minute and 9 at five minutes. There was a maternal history of spina bifida. A defect over the lumbar-sacral area was noted at delivery.

The patient was transferred, on the day of birth, to neonatologists at the University Children's Hospital at Hermann from another Texas hospital for evaluation and surgery. The myelomeningocele was surgically closed shortly after hospital admission. During the course of a 2-week hospitalization, evaluation revealed five major medical problems: (1) lumbar meningomyelocele, (2) gastrointestinal reflux, (3) renal disorder, (4) orthopedic abnormality (club feet), and (5) neurologic dysfunction secondary to Arnold-Chiari malformation and aqueductal stenosis. The head size progressively increased, and brain CT and ultrasound confirmed hydrocephalus (see Figure 12.4).

Initial ABR measurements were made on the fourth day of life. As shown in Figure 12.5 (top waveform), a reliable ABR was recorded and major wave components were observed. However, both caudal (I–III) and rostral (III–V) brain stem transmission times were markedly prolonged, even when interpreted according to age-matched normative data. Based on clinical findings, radiography, and these ABR data, a ventriculo-peritoneal shunt procedure was performed two weeks later. One day after the shunt procedure, brain stem transmission times were within age-corrected normal limits. Wave I was also larger. One week after surgery, the patient was discharged with normal mental development, although ataxic movements were observed, as well as paralysis of foot movement.

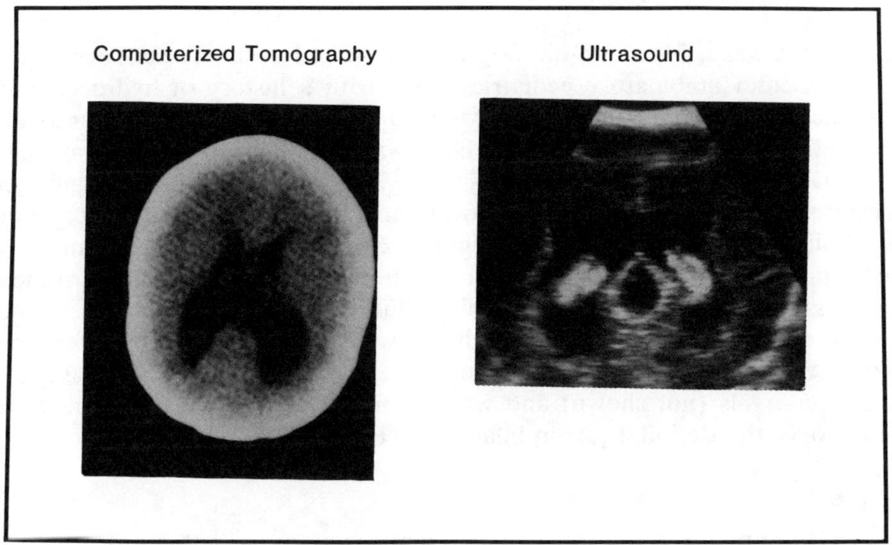

Figure 12.4   CT and ultrasound images for a newborn infant with hydrocephalus (case 3).

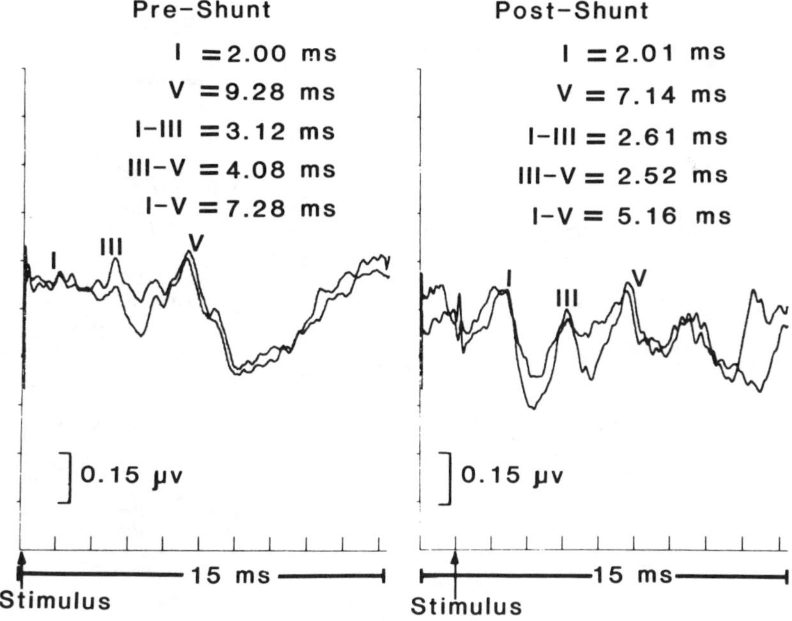

Figure 12.5   Auditory brain stem response (ABR) recordings before and after ventriculo-peritoneal shunt procedure for case 3. Waveforms are for right ear stimulation. ABR data were symmetrical.

Case 4. VERs in Hydrocephalus

The patient was a 21-month-old boy who presented at the Texas Tech Health Science Center ambulatory pediatrics clinic with a history of hydrocephalus. Examination of serial CT scans showed no significant changes in ventricular size, but by the mother's report the child was beginning to demonstrate signs of ataxia and irritability. SER assessment yielded a mild delay in brain stem transmission times by ABR (not shown) and VER waveforms of very poor morphology and small amplitude (Figure 12.6). The patient was admitted to the hospital and underwent surgery for insertion of a right ventriculo-peritoneal, low-pressure shunt. Clear cerebral spinal fluid under high pressure was noted to flow well when a ventricular catheter was placed in the right ventricle. Repeat SER assessment the following day showed normal ABR wave I–V latency intervals (not shown) and well-formed VER cortical components recorded over the occipital region bilaterally (Figure 12.6).

Comments

Cases 3 and 4 illustrate the application of SERs in managment of hydrocephalus, a topic that has attracted increased attention in recent years [4,10,17–19]. Both the ABR and VER can play an important role in early detection of the extent

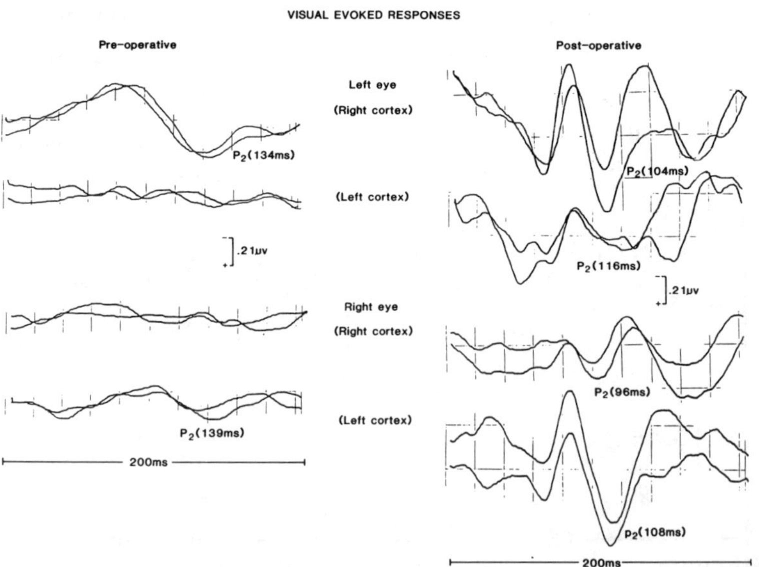

Figure 12.6 Visual evoked response waveforms before and after ventriculo-peritoneal shunt procedure of a 21-month-old boy with acute hydrocephalus (case 4).

of serious brain dysfunction and in documenting the effectiveness of surgical therapy. SERs, moreover, can be reliably recorded serially at bedside, or in the operating room, even from neonates and young children [9]. The ABR, in addition, provides a means of early detection of peripheral auditory deficits that may result from hydrocephalus in up to 25% of acute cases [10].

DISCUSSION

For over a decade, SERs have been applied in the ICU setting with adult populations [1]. Our experience [6,7,12], and that of others [2–4, 8, 9, 11, 13, 18, 20, 21], indicates that SERs are also a feasible means of assessing CNS status of children who have diverse acute brain pathology. SER measurement uniquely supplements the traditional bases of clinical data available for monitoring the acutely brain-injured child and is especially valuable as an early index of brain ischemia [12–15] in patients whose medical therapy (e.g., neuromuscular blocking agents, sedatives, barbiturates) precludes valid clinical neurologic examination [20–22].

Analyses of group findings would suggest that SERs are correlated with routinely monitored clinical parameters, such as pupillary response, blood pressure, ICP, and blood gases. In some cases, SERs do offer neurophysiologic confirmation of specific CNS pathophysiology. However, as illustrated by the case reports, marked discrepancies between SER results and these clinical findings may occur. For example, patients with CNS structural integrity, as reflected by unremarkable CT scans, may in fact have distinct deficits in neural function, as reflected by abnormal SERs. We have repeatedly observed acceptable ICP values monitored in patients with absent SER cortical components. Conversely, we have recorded SERs of normal latency and amplitude from patients with CT evidence of transtentorial herniation or fixed and dilated pupils [4,23,24].

It appears that SER findings complement general physiologic monitors and structural evidence of brain injury (CT, ultrasound). Reliance on a battery of independent parameters of neuronal structure and function probably offers the only valid and consistently accurate measure of CNS status. As a component in this test battery, SERs can contribute to medical decisions in the pediatric ICU, and can be applied in evaluating the effectiveness of medical and surgical therapy.

ACKNOWLEDGMENT

We gratefully acknowledge the assistance of Judy Mackey-Hargadine, M.D. (subject selection), and June Amling, R.N., M.S. (data analysis).

REFERENCES

1. Aguilar EA, Hall JW, Mackey-Hargadine JR. Neuro-otologic evaluation of the acute severely head-injured patient: Correlation among physical findings, auditory evoked responses and computerized tomography. Otolaryngol Head Neck Surg 1986;94:211–19.
2. Goitein K, Fainmesser P, Sohmer H. Cerebral perfusion pressure and auditory brain-stem responses in childhood CNS diseases. Am J Physiol 1983;137:777–81.
3. Greenberg RP, Becker DP, Miller JD, Mayer DJ. Evaluation of brain function in severe head trauma with multimodality evoked potentials. II. Localization of brain dysfunction in correlation with post-traumatic neurologic conditions. J Neurosurg 1977;47:163–77.
4. Guthkelch AN, Sclabassi RJ, Vries JK. Changes in the visual evoked potentials of hydrocephalic children. Neurosurgery 1982;11:599–602.
5. Hall JW. The effects of high-dose barbiturates on acoustic reflexes and auditory evoked responses. Acta Otolaryngol 1985;100:387–98.
6. Hall JW, Mackey-Hargadine JR, Kim EE. Auditory brainstem response (ABR) in determination of brain death. Arch Otolaryngol 1985;111:613–20.
7. Hall JW, Tucker DA. Sensory evoked responses in the intensive care unit. Ear Hearing 1986;7:220–32.
8. Hecox KE, Cone B. Prognostic importance of brainstem auditory evoked responses after asphyxia. Neurology 1981;31:1429–34.
9. Kraus N, Ozdamar O, Heydemann PT, Stein L, Reed NL. Auditory brainstem responses in hydrocephalic patients. Electroencephalogr Clin Neurophysiol 1984;59:310–31.
10. Lesnick JE, Michele JJ, Simeone FA, DeFeo S, Welsh FA. Alteration of somatosensory evoked potentials in response to global ischemia. J Neurosurg 1984;60:490–94.
11. Lütschg J, Pfenninger J, Ludin HP, Fassela F. Brain-stem auditory evoked potentials and early somatosensory evoked potentials in neurointensively treated comatose children. Am J Physiol 1983;137:421–26.
12. Mackey-Hargadine JR, Hall JW. Sensory evoked responses in head injury. Cent Nerv Sys Trauma 1985;2:187–206.
13. McPherson DL, Amlie R, Foltz E. Auditory brainstem responses in infant hydrocephalus. Childs Nerv Sys 1985;1:70–76.
14. Nagao S, Sunami N, Tsutsui T, Honma T, Doi A, Nishimoto A. Serial observations of brain stem function by auditory brain stem responses in central transtentorial herniation. Surg Neurol 1982;17:355–57.
15. Newlon PG, Greenberg RP, Hyatt MS, Enas GG, Becker DP. The dynamics of neuronal dysfunction and recovery following severe head injury assessed with serial multimodality evoked potentials. J Neurosurg 1982;57:168–77.
16. Nordby HK, Nesbakken R. The effect of high dose barbiturate decompression after severe head injury. A controlled clinical trial. Acta Neurochir 1984;72:157–66.
17. Samra SK, Krutak-Krol H, Pohorecki R, Domino EF. Scopolamine, morphine and brain-stem auditory evoked potentials in awake monkeys. Anesthesiology 1985;62:437–41.

18. Sklar FH, Ehle AL, Clark WK. Visual evoked potentials: A noninvasive technique to monitor patients with shunted hydrocephalus. Neurosurgery 1979;4:529–34.
19. Sohmer H, Gafni M, Chisin R. Auditory nerve-brain stem potentials in man and cat under hypoxic and hypercapnic conditions. Electroencephalogr Clin Neurophysiol 1982;53:506–12.
20. Stockard JE, Stockard JJ, Kleinber F, Westmoreland BF. Prognostic value of brainstem auditory evoked potentials in neonates. Arch Neurol Psychiatry 1983;40:360–65.
21. Strickbine-Van Reet P, Glaze DG, Hrachovy RA. A preliminary prospective neurophysiological study in children. Am J Physiol 1984;138:492–95.
22. Sutton LN, Bruce DA, Welsh F. The effect of cold-induced brain edema and white-matter ischemia on the somatosensory evoked response. J Neurosurg 1980;53:180–84.
23. Yagi T, Baba N. Evaluation of the brain-stem function by the brainstem response and the caloric vestibular reaction in comatose patients. Arch Otorhinolaryngol 1983;238:33–43.
24. York DH, Pulliam MW, Rosenfeld JG, Watts C. Relationship between visual evoked potentials and intracranial pressure. J Neurosurg 1981;55:909–16.

Part IV

Resources, Economics, and Malpractice

Karen A. Wagner

As the sheer number of survivors of head injury increases, factors that previously had minimal societal impact begin to demand attention. Manpower, hospital, and financial resource availability appear to be behind the advances in technology. Professor Bryan Jennett discusses the attempts being made to arrive at a better understanding of the problem of resource allocation. The economic impact of the long-term program of caring for and rehabilitating survivors is detailed in Mark Johnston's work. The notion of cost-effectiveness and cost-benefit must be considered from many perspectives. Cost in the financial sense and in the sense of the personal costs are both borne by survivors, their families, and friends throughout the life-long recovery process. Yet, even with these economic concerns, the pressure continues for the provision of the highest technological level of medical care within the hospital trauma centers. The issues in establishing medical malpractice in this super-specialized arena of medicine are presented by Robert Rand. In closing this section, Mitchell Rosenthal reviews past research in the rehabilitative care of the survivors of traumatic brain injury. A much speeded pace for future research efforts is demanded by the tremendous need for the resolution of the thirteen problem areas that he specifies.

Chapter 13

Resource Allocation for the Care of Head Injuries

Bryan Jennett

Accidents are now the leading cause of death in persons under the age of 45 years in westernized countries. Even in Third World countries in persons aged 5 to 45 years, accidents loom larger than any single disease classified by the World Health Organization. Brain injuries account for 70% of accidental deaths and in the United Kingdom for 15% of all deaths in persons aged 5 to 35 years. In the United States, brain injuries account for over half of all deaths in the age group 5 to 14 years, 70% of deaths between 15 and 24 years, and 62% of deaths between 25 and 34 years. Accidents account for many years of potential life lost—more than those from all types of cancer and heart disease together. More important still, brain injuries are a major cause of lifelong disability. Recovery after other types of trauma is usually good; only when the brain or spinal cord is damaged does permanent handicap result. Head injuries are 10 times more frequent than spinal injuries which, however, tend to be more visible in their residual disability and to attract more sympathy and attention. The average age of brain-injured survivors is about 27 years, and they may therefore face an average of 30 to 40 years of disability. There are now estimated to be as many persons neurologically disabled due to brain injury as due to stroke in the United Kingdom, where less than half as many head injuries occur as in the United States, but where the incidence of stroke is similar.

Another feature of head injury is that damage to the brain is frequently not maximal at onset. Instead, injury often sets in motion certain progressive pathological processes. Management is mainly directed toward anticipating, recognizing, and dealing adequately with these secondary complications. Outcome therefore often depends on the right action being taken at the right time, in the right place, and by the right person. The important challenges that head injuries present to the health care system of a developed country are that they are so common, that most victims are young, and that appropriate management can crucially affect the outcome.

Some 15 years ago in Glasgow we coined a phrase about head-injured patients who "talk and die." The implication was that a patient who had talked should not have died [1]. Such patients comprised a third of patients in neurosurgical units in more than one region of Britain 10 to 15 years ago. Autopsy of several hundred such cases in the Glasgow neurosurgical unit revealed that most had evidence of having had an increase in intracranial pressure, most had had hypoxic brain damage, and three fourths had had an intracranial hematoma removed. This led us to explore the incidence of avoidable factors contributing to the death of head-injured persons who had been hospitalized. We classified avoidable factors according to what went wrong, and where and when this had happened [2]. Was it delay in diagnosis or treatment, or were the measures simply inadequate? Did the fault occur at the roadside, in the ambulance, at the first hospital, or later? Delay in the diagnosis and evacuation of intracranial hematoma proved to be the most frequent avoidable factor. Next was impaired cerebral oxygenation, usually caused by a combination of systemic hypotension and hypoxia with raised intracranial pressure. That, in turn, frequently resulted from insufficient appreciation of the need, when there are multiple injuries, to give priority to the diagnosis of significant extracranial injuries. Carrying out initial resuscitation and treatment for these injuries is essential to protect the brain from further damage.

Several pertinent questions arise about those who have died after head injury. Were all deaths at the scene or on arrival at the hospital inevitable? Were all deaths in those who talked and died avoidable? When death was postponed by aggressive early care and subsequent support, was the large expenditure of effort and resources justified? In the United States and Australia, about two thirds of deaths occur before the patient reaches hospital, but in the United Kingdom the proportion is now only just over 40%. Analysis suggests that few could have been saved by expert interventions at the scene because most had overwhelming brain damage, a dislocated cervical spine or massive intrathoracic injury, or a combination of these. Diverting large resources toward elaborate roadside care may therefore be unwise.

Head-injured persons in the community as a whole, as opposed to those who find their way to university neurosurgical units, comprise a large and complex group of patients. Indeed, the pervasive nature of the head injury problem, straddling as it does a spectrum from the scene of the accident to persisting disability, accounts for why the care provided is often unsatisfactory. The dispersion of patients with head injury among so many disciplines in medicine and its associated health care professions makes their management difficult, and it raises the question "who cares for head injuries?" [3]. Where should resources go? To paramedics at the roadside, to emergency rooms, to primary hospitals dealing with less severe injuries, to intensive management of the severely brain damaged, or to the rehabilitation of survivors? Focus on costs and benefits might lead to a different balance in the distribution of resources than prevails at present.

Concern with this issue led us to set up the Scottish Head Injury Management Study in 1974 to survey all cases of head injury across the country.

It was followed by a series of epidemiological studies in several parts of the United States and in two states in Australia. The Scottish study remains the only one that is comprehensive, in the sense that it deals with injuries of all severities—from early deaths in persons who do not get to the hospital, to attenders at emergency rooms who are sent home [4]. As there are more than five times as many of the latter as are admitted to hospital, it is clear that the neurosurgeon sees only a minority of the patients who reach the hospital after head injury.

This is particularly so in European countries and in Australia—indeed in most countries other than the United States, which alone has enough neurosurgeons for most large community hospitals to have one on their staff. Most other countries depend on regional neurosurgical units, and the question of triage then occurs at two levels. The first is whether to admit a patient from the emergency room to a surgical bed in a primary hospital; the second is to decide which of these patients should then be transferred to a neurosurgical unit for special investigation and care, either directly or after further observation. However, it seems that although many community hospitals in the United States claim to have a neurosurgeon on their staff, this does not imply that a fully trained neurosurgical team is standing by 24 hours a day, as would be the case in a European regional neurosurgical unit. Whereas other countries are concerned with delay in referral from primary hospitals to neurosurgeons, in the United States delays can occur while waiting for a neurosurgeon to visit the community hospital at the end of a busy day in the main hospital miles away. Consider this statement last year from the declaration of the California Association of Neurosurgeons: "Amid this plethora of interest groups stand the neurosurgeons, few in number but crucial. The neurosurgeon knows what constitutes quality neurosurgical care for trauma . . . and that he cannot be in two hospitals at once" [5].

The same month as this statement was published, the American College of Surgeons published their *Document on Resources for Trauma Care,* with an appendix on neurotrauma approved by the AANS and CNS [6]. From a European perspective, it seems that the United States is moving toward regionalized neurosurgical centers for serious head injuries, including those deemed at risk of becoming serious from predictable complications. What a European has to say about the state of head injury care may therefore be more relevant for the next decade in America than it would have been for the last.

There is a difference in the rate of occurrence of head injuries. They occur more than twice as often in the United States, in Canada, in Australia, and in most European countries as they do in gentler countries such as the United Kingdom, Scandinavia, and Japan. These comparisons are based on death rates, the measure of brain injury incidence that is least open to administrative manipulation or differences in health care systems. However, the ratio between the number of patients admitted and the number who die varies widely between countries. This may reflect a difference in either the pattern of injury or the pattern of care. It could be that fewer mild injuries occur in America, but it seems more likely that American emergency room doctors admit many fewer mild injuries than do their counterparts in the United Kingdom. This might seem surprising in view of the legal harassment of American doctors, but the reason may be that many more U.S. primary hospitals have CT scanners as well as neurosurgical residents to screen patients in emergency rooms before they are sent home. The number of admissions in Britain is now decreasing as a result of guidelines that recommend that fewer mild injuries need to be admitted for observation.

Publicity often implies that road accidents are the main cause of head injury. This is not so even in the United States and Australia, where less than half the serious or fatal injuries are the result of road accidents. We have found that the distribution of causes varies widely according to severity of injury. In Scotland, among persons who arrive at emergency rooms after recent head injuries but are sent home, twice as many have had alcohol-related falls or assaults as road accidents. Another myth is that trauma is a growing epidemic. That is true only for developing countries as they simultaneously increase their consumption of alcohol and gasoline, which can be a fatal combination. In westernized countries, deaths from all accidents, including brain injuries, have been steadily decreasing in the last decade, and in the United Kingdom since 1968. The main reasons are preventive measures on the road, in industry, and in sports.

Planning the allocation of resources for the care of head injuries in a community has to take account of these various epidemiological features as they apply locally. Resources should be directed to minimizing avoidable death and disability, which applies whether a head injury is mild or severe. Most overall benefit is likely to come from reducing the risk of secondary brain damage by better management of complications in less severe injuries. We must therefore ensure that an appropriate proportion of resources do go to the prediction, prevention, detection, and treatment of these secondary events.

Methods and management objectives differ for patients with injuries of different severity. How severe an injury is may be judged when they present in the emergency room, or after hospital admission, and this judgment can be refined by using the Glasgow Coma Score. When this score was used to give three grades of severity, the proportions in the severe category in Edinburgh, Scotland, in Charlottesville, Virginia, and in Sydney, Australia, were 5%, 21%, and 10%, respectively [7–9]. These proportions are important because they suggest how resources should be distributed. Only a minority of patients are in the severe group that obviously need the skills of neurosurgeons. More overall benefit might result if more attention were paid to the less severely injured patients, because their outcome may be more readily influenced. Most instances of avoidable mortality and morbidity occur in these patients, as evidenced from analysis of "talk and die" patients. Moreover, because of their large numbers these less severely injured persons constitute most of the patients with intracranial hematoma, most of those requiring intracranial surgery, and most of those who are left with significant disability after the acute stage is over.

However, it would be a waste of expensive and limited resources to have large numbers of mild head injuries treated in major neurosurgical units. A reasonable policy should be devised that ensures that as few patients as possible will be at risk from avoidable mortality and morbidity. The rational response to this challenge is for neurosurgeons to analyze the diagnostic, monitoring, and therapeutic needs of various kinds of head-injured patients. Then they should consider which patients are sufficiently dependent on neurosurgical facilities to justify their being admitted to a neurosurgical service. Systematic statistical analysis is required to establish prognostic factors, such as which mildly injured patients are likely to develop complications, and which severely injured patients are retrievable. The aim is to apply triage in order to concentrate efforts on those patients whose outcome depends on different facilities and procedures. The way in which this is done will vary in different countries, but the principles are the same.

We have reviewed large numbers of patients both in accident/emergency rooms and in primary surgical wards to establish the risk that an intracranial hematoma will develop in patients who are talking and walking. These are patients likely to be sent home except for this risk [10]. Two factors are of prime importance: whether there is any impairment of consciousness, and whether there is a skull fracture. Given only these two readily available items of data it is possible to range the risks in different patients from 1 in 6,000 to 1 in 4. What level of risk calls for what level of provision of facilities, and at what level of accessibility or availability, will depend on local geography and on health care resources.

In the United Kingdom, guidelines were published based on discussion among 15 neurosurgeons from different parts of the country [11]. These defined criteria for skull x-ray in the emergency room, for admission to primary surgical wards, and for neurosurgical consultation and transfer. The Glasgow Institute has summarized these on a plastic card and distributed copies to all 21 referring hospitals in its region. Since the guidelines were published, admission rates to surgical wards in several parts of the country have been markedly reduced, and transfers to neurosurgical units have increased; this implies a significant shift in the distribution of resources. Twice as many brain injuries are now transferred each year to the Glasgow unit, where they account for significantly more bed days than previously. An essential part of this policy is that patients are returned to less expensive general surgical wards as soon as they no longer require the services of the neurosurgical unit. Based on such a policy we have calculated the number of beds, per million population, required to enforce the guidelines [12].

Too often the point of discharge from the neurosurgical unit marks the end of the clinical triumph over the immediate threat of death and the beginning of a lingering war of attrition for a patient and family against lifelong disability. Neurosurgeons need to examine the sense of devoting unlimited expenditure at the acute stage in order to secure survival, but then leaving the provision of adequate continuing care to chance. It is difficult to know how much should be spent in the rehabilitation phase to try to reduce the risks of secondary psychosocial morbidity in both the patient and the family. The evidence shows that recovery is extremely slow and very limited after a year and that family stresses actually get worse over the next few years. People tend not to adapt to the brain-injured survivor, and their sympathy and tolerance begin to flag. There are tough decisions to be made, including distinguishing between active rehabilitation on the one hand and long-term care for the patient and support of the family on the other. Rehabilitation using skilled personnel is expensive; it must be carefully considered how much of an investment in that, as distinct from the provision of social support, is worthwhile.

Because so much is spent on the management of head injury, it is important to discover whether the neurosurgeon's self-defined objective of reducing avoidable mortality and morbidity is being achieved. That calls for ongoing audit, year by year, for which the denominator should be the community rather than the selected subset of patients who are referred to a tertiary facility. What matters is whether an adequate service is being provided to the community in that as many appropriate patients as possible are gaining access to necessary facilities and are receiving effective treatment once they get there.

A more difficult matter is whether various regimens of management deliver reasonable value for money. How should we count the cost? Is it per day or per case? Or are we willing to be realistic and count the cost of success [13]? The cost of a survivor comprises not only the dollar costs of treatment in intensive care but also the cost of failing to save the two or three other patients whose treatment continued for a time even after it had become obvious that the outlook was hopeless. This estimate of cost will be influenced by how success is measured—in particular, how quality of life is judged for patients with persisting disability [14]. This has not been done for head injury, but an example from neonatal intensive care indicates the principle. The triumphs of salvaging low-birth-weight babies are bought at the price of nonsurvivors whose treatment usually costs more than that of the survivors [13]. Indeed, the cost of securing a survivor among the lower-weight babies who have a worse prognosis is twice that of the bigger babies. When the number of life years gained is counted, the difference in cost is three times greater for smallerbabies. If the poor quality of life in some survivors is allowed for when calculating the cost per quality-adjusted life year (QALY), then the cost of securing a QALY by treating the lower-birth-weight babies is seven times greater. How would such an analysis look for the management of brain injuries of varying severity with varying levels of disability in survivors?

Do we take sufficient care not only to avoid inappropriate expenditure but also to think about how unkind this can sometimes be? In particular, do we face up to decisions about appropriate management of hopeless patients, especially now that reliable statistical predictions can often be made that patients will not survive, or if they do that they cannot make reasonable recoveries? It is the expense of prolonged dying or of survival in a vegetative state that no country can afford, either financially or in humanitarian terms. If we wasted fewer resources in this way we could afford more of the expensive successes.

Finally, do we invest enough in research, particularly in clinical research on evaluating the expensive management we provide? In the computing, defense, and pharmaceutical industries some 10 to 12% of expenditures goes to research and development [15]. But only 3% goes to research and development in health care delivered at the bedside in the United States, and this is less than it was 10 years ago. In my view as an academic clinician, clinical research is where we need more effort, and it will eventually result in better and more cost-effective patient care.

REFERENCES

1. Reilly PL, Graham DI, Adams JH, Jennett B. Patients with head injury who talk and die. Lancet 1975;2:375–77.
2. Rose J, Valtonen S, Jennett B. Avoidable factors contributing to death after head injury. Br Med J 1977;2:615–18.
3. Jennett B. Who cares for head injuries? Br Med J 1975;3:267–70.
4. Jennett B, MacMillan R. Epidemiology of head injuries. Br Med J 1981;282:101–4.
5. Smith RW. Guidelines for establishment of trauma centers. J Neurosurg 1986;65:569–71.
6. Anonymous. Planning neurotrauma care. (Appendix 1 to the Hospital Resources Document). Am Coll Surg Bull 1986;71:22–23.
7. Miller JD, Jones PA. The work of a regional head injury service. Lancet 1985;1:1141–44.
8. Jagger J, Levine JI, Jane JA, Rimel RW. Epidemiologic features of head injury in a predominately rural population. J Trauma 1984;1:40–44.
9. Lyle DM, Pierce JP, Freeman EA. Clinical course and outcome of severe head injury in Australia. J Neurosurg 1986;65:15–18.
10. Mendelow AD, Teasdale G, Jennett B, Bryden J, Hessett C, Murray G. Risks of intracranial hematoma in head injured adults. Br Med J 1983;287:1173–76.
11. A group of neurosurgeons. Guidelines for initial management after head injury in adults. Br Med J 1984;288:983–85.
12. Bryden J, Jennett B. Neurosurgical resources and transfer policies for head injuries. Br Med J 1983;286:1791–93.
13. Jennett B. High technology medicine. Benefits and burdens. 2nd ed. New York: Oxford University Press, 1986.
14. Jennett B. High technology medicine and the quality of life. Int J Tech Assess Health Care 1987;3:51–60.
15. Jennett B. Assessment of medical technologies. Lancet 1986;2:735–36.

Chapter 14

The Economics of Brain Injury: A Preface

Mark V. Johnston

Although substantial progress has been made in recent years in improving survival after brain injury, in developing systems of rehabilitative care for brain-injured persons, and in understanding epidemiology and prognosis, little work has been published regarding the economics of brain injury. It is known that traumatic brain injuries (TBI) are a common cause of hospitalization, and it is logical to deduce that they inflict substantial economic losses on the country. But estimates of the size of economic losses vary enormously. The National Head and Spinal Cord Injury Survey (NHSCI) [1] estimated nationwide costs due to traumatic brain injury (TBI) as $3.9 billion annually, whereas Grabow et al [2] estimated costs as $12.5 billion.

The economics of brain injury encompass more than dollar costs. One must ask whether proposed interventions save lives and avert suffering, for it is precisely in the improvement of human lives that the economic utility of interventions lies. From an economic perspective, the benefits of any intervention need to be balanced against the costs, which represent increased burdens to other human beings. Monetary figures are a convenient but incomplete way of summarizing these tradeoffs.

Little has been published directly on the cost-benefits or cost-effectiveness of alternative ways of dealing with problems in brain injury. However, a great deal of work can be found in closely related areas.

THE SCOPE OF THE PROBLEM

Approximately half a million persons are hospitalized each year in the United States for TBI. According to the National Head and Spinal Cord Injury Survey of 1970 to 1974, about 422,000 of these were initial hospitalizations [1,3]. This implies an incidence rate of about 200 first hospitalizations per 100,000 population. These figures compare with about 10,000 hospitalizations for spinal cord injury (SCI), or a rate of 5 per 100,000. The rate of hospitalization for TBI is about 40 times as great as that for SCI, a type of injury for which rehabilitation and disability care systems are much more highly developed.

Interviews of the general population report substantially larger numbers of brain injuries than those found from hospital records. For instance, the U.S. Health Interview Survey of 1975 reported 1,408,000 brain injuries, including 613,000 concussions and 663,000 unspecified brain injuries [4]. If only half of these involved common criteria for TBI (loss of consciousness, postraumatic amnesia, or skull fracture), the total incidence rate of TBI would be about 300 per 100,000 population.

About 3% of those hospitalized for TBI (about 12,660 persons) die from their injuries [3]. However, about 70,000 persons die annually from TBI before reaching the hospital [5]. A fatality rate of 11.65% (35/270 males, 10/116 females) was found in patients within 28 days of injury in Olmsted County, Minnesota from 1965 to 1974 [6]; this rate declined to 9.2% in a cost study for 1970 to 1974 (J. D. Grabow, unpublished data, 1987). Field [7] found that 60% of deaths due to brain injury occurred before hospital admission. Jennett [8] reports that the United States suffers 22 to 25 fatal brain injuries per 100,000 population —a rate about twice that of Japan, the United Kingdom, or Sweden. Kraus's review [5] of five population-based studies indicates that age-adjusted fatality rates for TBI ranged from 22 to 30 per 100,000 persons in the United States, or 51,000 to 71,000 deaths annually.

It is well known that TBI occurs most frequently among persons aged 15 to 24 years but is almost as frequent among younger persons. Of all persons hospitalized for TBI, 63% are less than 25 years old [3]. More than twice as many males incur TBI as females. Approximately 49% of brain injury hospitalizations are due to automobile or motorcycle accidents; another 28% are due to falls, and about 22% are due to drug overdoses, guns, anoxia, or other causes [1,3]. The rate of anoxic and chemical brain damage has been underestimated or not estimated at all in most studies of brain injury.

Disability Produced by TBI

There are no accurate figures, nationally or regionally, on the extent of disability produced by TBI [5]. The absence of such data is a critical barrier to better understanding of the economics of TBI. The best available sources indicated that about 10 to 18% of persons with mild brain injuries are left with some disability (Glasgow Coma Scale [GCS] greater than 11; 32,000 to 56,600 persons annually); two-thirds of moderately brain-injured persons are left with some disability (GCS 8 to 11; 24,924 persons annually); and 100% of severely brain-injured persons sustain long-term disabilities (GCS less than 8; 16,800 annually) [5]. Between 73,724 and 98,325 persons would then be disabled annually by TBI. The duration of disability for these persons is not clear. It is estimated that about 2,000 persons annually remain in coma or persistent vegetative state [9,10].

These expert judgments, based on extrapolation from studies in various regions, are useful, but precise estimates based on random sampling of the population would be much preferable. Long-term follow-up of a representative cohort of brain-injured persons at all levels of severity is especially needed, but there are no such studies in the United States.

It is generally accepted that advances in neurotrauma treatment have led to an increasing number of persons who survive severe brain injury but are left severely disabled. It is widely believed that the incidence of TBI has increased in recent decades. Although it is not clear that this increase has continued into the 1980s, there are still strong reasons to believe that the population of persons disabled by TBI is increasing rapidly.

Effects of TBI on Employment

Lost earnings are by far the largest economic cost associated with TBI. Computation of lost earnings is essential in estimating the costs of TBI and the benefits of interventions to alleviate problems associated with TBI.

Table 14.1 summarizes the results of ten studies of unemployment and long-term disability for TBI survivors. From these figures it is clear that most persons hospitalized for TBI return to work in a few days or weeks. But there is an increase in the unemployment rate of between 10 and 20% for many years, even decades, after the injury.

A more precise summary of the information awaits further study. Future research should present results in a form that permits comparison with other studies. Results need to be stratified according to severity of injury. Longitudinal studies portraying the decrease in employment over several years, as well as retrospective studies with good case-finding methods, are needed. Unemployment figures need to be compared with those for the local population or a control group (e.g., one matched on job skills, education, age, and gender) to be valid for economic analysis. Estimates of monetary earnings need to be reported.

NATIONWIDE COSTS OF BRAIN INJURY

Two estimates of the nationwide costs of brain injury have been published. The first comes from the National Head and Spinal Cord Injury Survey, which sampled patients discharged from American hospitals during the years 1970 through 1974 [1,3]. Inflating to 1980 price levels, they estimated direct costs of TBI to be $1.14 billion annually. Direct costs are expenses incurred directly for medical care, equipment, hospitalization (the largest component of direct costs), and so on. Indirect costs were much larger: $2.76 billion dollars annually; these were defined as losses due to restricted productivity (lost earnings) in the patient or family or friends. Total nationwide costs (direct and indirect combined) were estimated at $3.9 billion annually.

The second study giving estimates of nationwide costs is particularly good because it is a study of a full population rather than hospital cases alone. Grabow et al [2] obtained information on virtually all cases of brain injury that

Table 14.1 Unemployment Following Traumatic Brain Injury

Study	Unemployment Rates[a]	Time Postinjury	Comments
Jane et al [11]	34% for mild TBI	3 mo	Referrals to University of Virginia, including cases with alcohol involvement and previous TBI
Wagner [12]	10% for mild TBI 20% for moderate TBI 57% for severe TBI	2 yrs	In Houston, 1982–1984
Dresser et al [13]	20% greater than a control group	15 yrs	U.S. veterans; control group of veterans similar in age, rank, unit, and time of service
Gilchrist and Wilkinsen [14]	59%; severe cases	9 mo–15 yrs	n = 84 younger cases in London from 1963–1975
Brennan [15]	39% for severe TBI 12% for moderate & mild	9 mo	n = 296; in Ireland
Lewin et al [16]	At least 18% (4% totally disabled, 14% unable to engage in any normal occupation)	10 yrs	British; mortality rate > normal; 479 cases with at least 1 week of posttraumatic amnesia.
Oddy and Humphrey [17]	30% at 6 mo 17.8% at 1 yr 15.6% at 2 yrs	6 mo–2 yrs	Control group enemployment not reported
Brooks et al [18]	69%, severe cases	5 yrs	No increase in employment between 2 and 5 years
Prigatano et al [19]	38% for milder cases (GCS at acute hospital admission = 13–15) 50% for moderate (GCS = 9–12) 76% for severe (GCS = 8 or less)	2–4 yrs	Difficult to determine exact rates from publication
Jacobs [20]	80% among severe cases	1–6 yrs	Retrospective follow-up in Los Angeles

[a]Among survivors employed previous to the head injury.

came to medical or official attention in Olmsted County, Minnesota. Table 14.2 presents the Olmsted County data transformed to a cost-per-case basis by dividing by the number of cases. Three features of the table are worth emphasis. First, the largest component of total costs was lost lifetime earnings due to fatalities. Second, when averaged over all severity classes for the study year, earnings lost by patients ($110) were very slightly less than earnings lost by others ($118). The main reason for this was probably that many TBI patients were of school age, causing lost earnings to occur primarily to parents. Impact on the entire family must be measured to characterize the costs of TBI. Third, indirect costs of lost earnings averaged slightly higher for patients with "mild" head trauma than for those with "moderate" head trauma ($418 versus $269 per case). Such a finding raises the question of whether mild head injuries ("patients with loss of consciousness or posttraumatic amnesia of less than 30 minutes without skull fracture") are really mild. Research needs to develop improved criteria to classify severity of TBI.

Adjusting for differences in age and gender between Olmsted County and the nation, nationwide direct costs were estimated as $1.0 billion in 1982 price levels. Indirect costs were estimated as $11.5 billion, using a 6% discount rate. (The discount rate is the annual percentage by which future earnings are

Table 14.2 Estimated Average Costs per Case of Brain Trauma[a]

Costs	Mild	Moderate	Severe	Fatal
Direct	$1,031	$1,872	$16,260	$2,335
Indirect				
Lost income by patient	418	269	4,987	0
Lost income by others	139	794	6,158	0
Funeral	0	0	0	8,803
Subtotal	$558	$1,063	$11,145	$8,803
Present value of lifetime lost earnings at 6% discount rate				$256,285
Total indirect	$558	$1,063	$11,145	$265,087
Total, direct plus indirect	$1,589	$2,935	$27,405	$267,422
Average annual number of cases	103.4	43.6	11.0	16.2

[a]Recomputed from Grabow et al [2], Annegers et al [6], and unpublished data courtesy of J.D. Grabow, MD, February 1987. Cost figures inflated to 1982 price levels.

reduced to take into account the fact that money in the future is valued less than the same money today.)

The $1.0 billion estimate of direct costs is remarkably close to the $1.14 billion estimate of the NHSCI Survey. The small difference can be explained by the fact that the average cost of medical care in Olmsted County is somewhat less than that in the nation as a whole. But the $11.5 billion estimate for indirect costs is radically different from the $2.76 billion estimate of the NHSCI. What can account for such a discrepancy?

At first, one might suppose that the discrepancy is due to the fact that indirect costs, by nature, cannot be estimated as precisely as direct costs. However, the discrepancy here is too large to attribute to such natural ambiguities. The answer was found by meticulous reading of the two studies and perusal of unpublished background material: the NHSCI report did not project lifetime lost earnings but included only lost earnings during the study period. This method avoids uncertainties associated with projecting lifetime lost earnings, but does so by giving them a value of zero. Whatever the discount rate, it is certain that earnings losses do not cease at the end of the study but continue for decades into the future.

In contrast, the Olmsted County study attempted to follow patients for five years after their injury, and thus it includes a larger fraction of long-term losses. But even here, long-term losses in productivity appear to have been underestimated. If even 1 of the 11 annual severe patients had been permanently disabled, average indirect costs for the group would have exceeded $23,299 ($256,285/11); the average loss of income for the group ($4,987) appears to be too small.

An emphasis on losses due to mortality and an underestimate of losses due to morbidity is common in economic studies of the cost of illness (see, for example, Rice [2]). Morbidity losses due to TBI would tend to be underestimated using common methods that compute lost earnings on the basis of earnings for previously employed persons. Most brain injuries occur in younger persons who are unemployed, are students, or are in low-paying jobs at the beginning of their career. Application of the method to such persons excludes losses due to delay of employment, extended schooling and rehabilitation, lack of advancement, and failure by unemployed youths ever to obtain a job. This is a major problem. Remedies include comparison of unemployment rates and earnings with those in a similar control group and adjustment of raw averages on the basis of age, gender, and education.

In addition, economic losses can be even greater for permanently disabled persons than for fatalities, because lifetime care costs must be added to lost earnings. Currently available cost estimations do not take this into account.

A New Estimate of Nationwide Costs

It is not possible to correct existing estimates of nationwide TBI costs in any precise way. However, these estimates can be vastly improved by using reasonable approximations for previously omitted factors.

The first needed improvement involves estimation of the present value of lifetime lost earnings for fatalities. Such an estimate can be constructed using Kraus's [5] estimate of 70,000 annual TBI deaths and the Olmsted County estimate of $265,000 loss per fatality (see Table 14.2). Multiplying the two, one arrives at an estimate of $18.55 billion in annual losses due to fatalities. To apply this to the NHSCI data, one needs to add this figure to the $2.76 billion in indirect costs already documented in the NHSCI study and correct for one year of double counting of fatality losses (about $.79 billion). The resulting estimate for the indirect TBI costs is $20.52 billion.

Second, long-term costs incurred as a consequence of permanent disablement produced by TBI need to be estimated. The magnitude of such losses is particularly uncertain, but the studies reviewed above easily support estimates of lifetime increases in long-term unemployment rates in excess of 10% among previously employed, discharged TBI survivors. To be conservative, let us assume a 10% decrease in lifetime productivity among discharged TBI survivors. If one applies this assumption to the Olmsted County data, nationwide indirect costs due to long-term disability would be about $10.3 billion dollars. Adding long-term unemployment costs to other indirect costs from the Olmstead data (correcting for double count of 5 years), the total indirect cost of TBI would be about $22.8 billion. Adding long-term unemployment costs to the NHSCI figures (and correcting for the one-year double count) would give a cost of about $28.57 billion. Adjusting these figures for inflation to 1986 price levels yields estimates of $25.9 to $34.4 billion.

In sum, TBI appears to cost the United States approximately $25.9 to $34.4 billion annually in lost productivity. Although these estimates are much larger than previous ones, I do not believe that they are liberal, because long-term productivity losses due to reduced cognitive capacities and increased long-term support costs are not fully included here. At least another $1.86 billion is spent directly for medical care (inflating 1980 medical costs from the NHSCI to 1986 levels using the general rate of inflation of medical costs). This estimate, too, is conservative because it assumes that intensity of treatment for hospitalized TBI patients has not increased since 1974. More likely, intensity of treatment has increased substantially. A 50% increase in intensity would put 1986 direct medical costs at $2.79 billion. Empirical study of populations and follow-up studies that ask about loss of earnings are required to give more exact estimates.

ECONOMIC ISSUES AT THREE STAGES OF BRAIN INJURY

Although there is little research directly on the cost-effectiveness and cost-benefits of alternative interventions in TBI, we are far from ignorant of factors that affect cost-benefits and cost-effectiveness. Treatments and policies that are not effective cannot be cost-effective or cost-beneficial. Conversely, highly effective treatments and policies stand a good chance of being cost-effective;

even if they are not, ethical considerations may require that the treatment be provided anyway.

Prevention

Prevention is the only stage at which the entire $18 to $30 billion annual cost of TBI is relevant, for only prevention can totally avert costs of brain injury. There is a science of injury prevention just as surely as there is a science of medicine or rehabilitation [22].

Evidence of the effectiveness of seat belts, motorcycle helmets, physical changes in road design, signs, and other physical means of preventing injuries is overwhelming [23–25]. From the standpoint of social costs, substantial capital expenditures would be justified if they decreased the frequency of injuries. Assuming we demand a 10% return on investment, which is higher than the yield for current 30-year treasury bonds, an investment of $85 billion is justified if it averts just half ($8.5 billion) of the most conservative estimate of nationwide brain injury costs. Cost-benefits are a crucial issue, because eliminating some dangers can be very expensive (e.g., eliminating left turns by constructing overpasses).

Legislative interventions are undoubtedly effective in decreasing injuries. For example, the evidence for the effectiveness of motorcycle helmet laws is conclusive. In the 1970s, four states repealed laws requiring motorcycle helmet use [25]. In every state and by every index examined (number of accidents, number of fatalities, and duration of hospital stay), costs and severity of injuries increased. In Kansas there was a 189% increase in hospital costs for nonhelmeted drivers following repeal of helmet legislation. It should be noted that seat belt laws and the like are effective only with enforcement and public education.

Given the low cost and high effectiveness of legislative interventions, they are probably the most cost-effective and cost-beneficial means of lessening the costs of brain injury. The reason for opposition to laws requiring safe practice is not that there is any serious question of cost-benefits but that such laws conflict with American convictions regarding personal liberty. One of the most important current issues in prevention is how to increase the use of safety devices without resorting to legal sanctions [23]. Individual citizens need to understand the full long-run costs of dangerous behavior. At present the benefits of freedom, such as driving without seat belts, or earning profits from selling liquor to people who will need to drive home, are enjoyed by one group of individuals, whereas many of the costs are borne by others. These include higher taxes for Medicaid, higher insurance premiums paid by safe drivers, a shift in the bearing of private hospital costs to those with adequate insurance, and heavy burdens on the families of brain-injured persons. Freedom must be linked with responsibility.

Acute Medical Care

Treatment of TBI is a small part of medical care as a whole. Although a good deal of research has been done on cost control and cost effectiveness in the whole field of health care [26], it is unlikely that great resources will ever be devoted to economic analysis of TBI, per se. Most economic issues in the acute medical care of TBI are most fruitfully and practically approached as part of broader health care issues. Findings and principles in closely related areas should logically hold for brain injury as well.

Economics is based on the premise that resources are always limited. Cost-benefit analysis in management economics is based on computation of profit or loss under a set of assumptions or goals that include a fixed budget or other constraints [27]. Cost-benefit analysis is useless without economic incentives and without some administrative mechanism to make the ultimate limitations proximal: a budget.

In health care too, some definite means is required to limit expenditures and make decision makers face up to the reality of limited resources. The best example of this is prospective payment by Diagnostically Related Groups (DRGs), which sharply cut the rate of growth of Medicare hospital costs. DRGs are not the only ways to control costs. Health maintenance organizations (HMOs) can impose budgets based on capitation payment limits. Centralized socialized medicine systems can impose budgets. But without a budget, cost control is not possible and cost effectiveness is irrelevant. Efficient budgeting systems need to promote an internalized sense of what is worthwhile and what is wasteful among medical professionals, and to require that resource allocation decisions be made on the basis of this sense.

Clinical Issues

Clinical decisions in the medical care of TBI patients are fraught with economic implications, but only a few empirical studies can be found. For instance, one British study found that substantial sums could be saved if hospitals admitted fewer patients with histories of brief unconsciousness without skull fracture or other much more important risk factors following head injury [28]. Reiner et al provide evidence that selective peritoneal lavage in the management of comatose blunt trauma patients is more cost-beneficial than routine peritoneal lavage [29]. Bryan Jennett's chapter in this volume provides a more thorough treatment of economic issues in the acute medical care of TBI patients.

Coma and Persistent Vegetative State (PVS)

PVS differs from coma in that vegetative patients retain the capacity for subcortical responses such as open eyes, sleep-wake cycles, and startle reactions [30,31]. However, in both states psychologically meaningful responses, cognition of self or environment, and communication are not possible.

About 2,000 comatose patients are discharged from American hospitals each year (0.5% of hospital discharges [10] multiplied by the U.S. population). The number of institutional beds devoted to coma care has increased dramatically in recent years. Hospital care expenses for comatose patients range from $350 per day for simpler cases to $900 for many ventilator-dependent patients, excluding physician costs. Long-term maintenance costs for coma and PVS patients are much higher than for average nursing home patients. Charges of $350 to $500 per day are common. With good care, comatose or PVS patients will survive for years or even decades. Government (e.g., Medicaid) pays the majority of costs.

While most comatose TBI patients eventually recover to some degree, large numbers remain in coma or PVS until they die. Substantial resources continue to be devoted to PVS cases far beyond the point at which there is any realistic chance of recovery. Physicians have questioned "the utilization of precious resources for practices that benefit neither the individual nor society" [32]. More human good would be done by allocating therapeutic resources to persons more likely to benefit from them.

A less obvious economic issue is the need for high quality care and preventive rehabilitation for comatose patients who are likely to recover. Much coma care is of poor quality. Comatose patients develop complications that lead to expensive, recurrent hospital admissions. When patients finally begin to emerge from coma, acquired complications make their subsequent rehabilitation slower and more expensive.

The likelihood of recovery is critical to rational resource allocation in coma and PVS. Prognosis in coma and PVS is complex, and contradictory reports are frequently heard. One study found that among those patients remaining vegetative at three months postinjury, "the possibility of regaining an independent existence can be virtually excluded" [30]. In this study, 60% of patients in PVS at three months died within one year postinjury.

Though recovery of total independence is unlikely for many cases, recovery of some functional behavior is quite possible. A recent study found that 44% of brain injured patients who were totally lacking in any functional behavior at six months postonset regained some functional behavior with a long-term rehabilitative program [33]. Ten of 12 patients showing specific responses to stimuli at admission regained function, but only one of 10 cases lacking a pupillary light response did so.

The scientific literature on prognosis after coma/PVS exhibits both controversy and a trend toward increasing accuracy. Fifteen years ago, prognosis after severe brain injury was virtually impossible. Two years ago (1986), studies reported that the majority of patients for whom the likelihood of meaningful recovery is nil could be identified after one month in coma/PVS [30,31]. But even a small likelihood of a false negative (giving up on a patient who in fact would have improved) is unacceptable. That same year, an authoritative article concluded that physicians should wait one year postinjury to definitively diagnose persistent (i.e., permanent) vegetative state [31].

More recently, Giannotta et al [34] reported that prediction could be improved to a high degree of accuracy by using a range of predictors (age, GCS, pupillary reactions, oculocephalic reflex, and, especially, auditory evoked potentials) and combining them using log-linear techniques. Even though the prediction was made less than one week postinjury, it was 82% accurate in predicting recovery from PVS, and there were no false negatives in the prediction. Though these results need to be replicated in a larger sample, accurate prediction of recovery for most PVS patients appears to be just around the corner.

Attempts to legislate discontinuation of care for "hopeless" cases are morally repugnant. Legal interventions can increase costs by requiring continuation of treatment against the wishes of patient, family, and physician [35]. Leaving life support decisions as much as possible to those most intimately involved may be as economical as any other ethical policy in this country. At the same time, it is not unethical to ask that these persons face up to the social costs of their decisions. Case management and utilization review systems can be devised to save money and improve care by shifting resources away from comatose patients unlikely to recover toward those more likely to recover.

Rehabilitation

Although no exact figures are available, total expenditures for TBI rehabilitation are probably a small fraction of total direct TBI costs. However, data on costs per rehabilitation discharge are available. A recent survey conducted by Coopers and Lybrand for the National Association of Rehabilitation Facilities [36] reports an average length of stay of between 46 and 48 days (depending on the exact definition of "brain injury/damage") in American rehabilitation hospitals. Average length of stay was 38 to 39 days in the West and 49 to 52 in the central and eastern regions. Nationwide charges averaged $487 to $481 per day; costs per day, $357 to $353. Per day charges and costs were both higher in the West than elsewhere. A survey by the Rand Corporation done about the same time reported much shorter stay and lower charges [37], but the two studies agreed that there is great variation in length of stay and charges. The Rand study reported that about 25% of brain injury patients stayed in rehabilitation less than 15 days, whereas another 25% stayed in rehabilitation more than 55 days.

Cost-Effectiveness

Only two studies have been done on the cost effectiveness of head injury rehabilitation. Cope and Hall [38] found that patients admitted late to rehabilitation (greater than 35 days postinjury) required twice as much acute hospital care as those admitted earlier. The savings with earlier admission: $40,000 per case. The study is persuasive because early and late cases did not appear to differ in length of coma, age, or disability level. It is possible that the late group may have had other problems or medical complications that delayed referral to rehabilitation, but on balance the study provides evidence that early transfer of severe TBI cases to an organized acute brain injury rehabilitation unit was cost effective compared with continued treatment in less specialized hospital beds.

The second study, by Aronow, compared the outcomes of severe TBI survivors in California who received comprehensive rehabilitation with a group in Virginia who did not [39]. Aronow's study was hampered by the fact that the non-rehabilitation group was, on average, much less severely injured than the rehabilitation group. Matching and multiple regression were employed to alleviate this bias. Results after these statistical adjustments showed that rehabilitation appeared to have improved some outcomes. This improvement was statistically significant but small in magnitude. Two reasons for this result were evident. First, the effects of rehabilitation may be small or modest compared with the magnitude of effects produced by the brain injury. Second, the "noise" level in the study, that is, the amount of "error variance," was fairly great, making it difficult to detect real but less than dramatic effects.

Outcome data were translated into cost estimates. Comparing rehabilitated patients with non-rehabilitated patients with brain injury of similar severity, average annual savings of $11,949 were reported for rehabilitated patients with briefer posttraumatic amnesia (up to one month). Savings were much less for rehabilitated patients whose posttraumatic amnesia lasted longer. If these savings continue at the stated level after discharge, it would take only three years to recoup the cost of inpatient rehabilitation.

The statistical significance of the data on which these estimates were based was marginal, but the pattern of results is similar to that found in other studies of rehabilitation patients. A curvilinear relation between functional improvement and improvement per dollar has been reported for a variety of neurologically impaired rehabilitation patients [40–42]. The greatest improvement per dollar has most frequently been found for rehabilitation hospital inpatients with brain injury of intermediate severity. Improvement per dollar is frequently less for patients whose brain injury is of the greatest or the least severity.

The Need for Effectiveness Research

The most pressing priority in the study of the cost-benefits and cost-effectiveness of rehabilitation is better understanding of effectiveness. Without knowledge of which treatments or programs are effective, cost-benefits and cost-effectiveness cannot be estimated. The literature of rehabilitation provides a large number of studies that suggest that rehabilitation is effective and even cost-effective, but only a small number of studies are persuasive or conclusive (cf. Johnston and Keith [43]). Authoritative reviews of TBI rehabilitation have pled for better understanding of the processes underlying recovery and rehabilitation [44]. Demonstrating that patients improve during rehabilitation is not proof of effectiveness, for brain-injured persons can recover in the absence of professional rehabilitation. To prove that a rehabilitative intervention is effective, it is necessary to show that a patient group has improved more than it would have without such interventions.

In recent years, economic analysts in other areas of health care and in vocational rehabilitation have also become aware of the importance of controlled experiments. An example is Berkowitz's [45] analysis of the cost-benefit literature in vocational rehabilitation. Despite strenuous efforts to correct for problems, "None of these corrections . . . nor any we can think of, result in a benefit cost ratio in which we can have confidence." There were just too many uncertain parameters. However, "most of these problems would be minimal if we had a genuine control group or better longitudinal data."

Why has so little controlled research been done? Funding for rehabilitation research has never been great, and it has declined to less than half the level of the late 1960s [46]. According to one report, less than 0.2% of total federal expenditures for severely handicapped people is devoted to research and development [47]. Moreover, rehabilitation research is complex. Like other medical research, rehabilitation deals with impairments (problems at the organ system level). Yet it also deals with disabilities (life activities) and handicap (experiences that are the consequence of disabilities and impairments) [48,49]. Opportunities for ethical, controlled experimental research are rare and are difficult to implement.

But even in the absence of definitive studies, decisions about patients and funding must and will continue to be made. What is needed is to draw together what data exist and, on the basis of well-established principles, to reason about which rehabilitative strategies are likely to be more cost-effective and which are likely to be less so.

Cognitive Rehabilitation

Caplan [50] points out that there are a number of mechanisms by which cognitive rehabilitation might be effective: (1) reorganization within the brain by which undamaged portions acquire responsibility for performance; (2) substitution of a compensatory strategy based on residual functional capacities; and (3) minimizing the extent to which a patient's deficit impinges on daily life. There is controversy about which of these strategies is most effective, and judgments of the relative cost-effectiveness of these strategies would be premature.

However, discrepancies between the research literature and rehabilitative practices give us hints regarding practices that seem likely to be wasteful. One hears marketing personnel and more enthusiastic but less educated rehabilitation staff describe cognitive rehabilitation programs as if they aim at the direct restoration of dead neural structures (e.g., stimulation of dendritic growth). Respectable scientific works do not support the idea that TBI rehabilitation can be effective by direct restoration [51,52]. Treatment programs premised on direct restoration through practice are unlikely to be cost effective.

However, rehabilitation certainly involves learning. This is saying a lot, for we know a great deal about how learning works and how it does not in the disabled human brain (see, e.g., Matsun and McCartney [53]). For instance, generalization of skills to different situations is usually much more difficult to show than improvements in the target behavior. Evidence for the training of intelligence is scant compared with the great corpus of repeatedly validated results pertaining to methods of training skills or skill groups. Trauma restricts the brain's capacity to generalize. Training programs that assume that generalization will occur are unproven and are likely to be less cost effective than programs that train in needed skills and directly train for generalization. Thus, for instance, severely brain-injured persons can be trained to improve in memory and problem-solving tasks on a computer, but generalization of such skills to real-world problems has not been demonstrated.

Although memory problems of TBI individuals have been alleviated by environmental modifications (e.g., reminder systems) and by training in encoding and decoding strategies, there is no evidence that memory grows stronger from exercise or practice, per se [54]. Similarly, a recent study compared functional outcomes after discharge from an inpatient neuromuscular reeducation program to outcomes after traditional functional training program for stroke patients [55]. Functional outcomes eight months after discharge were virtually the same for the two therapeutic strategies, but costs were more than twice as great with neuromuscular reeducation (average length of stay = 68.3 versus 28.57 days). The sample size was small (20 and 19), and TBI differs from stroke. But the study certainly raises the question of whether neuromuscular reeducation and neurodevelopmental programming strategies are also less cost-effective than functional training in TBI rehabilitation.

Timing of Rehabilitation

There is evidence from animal studies that the level of recovery from brain injury depends on training or stimulation, and there is some preliminary evidence that recovery is somewhat greater if the training occurs shortly after the lesion rather than later [44]. The relevance of these findings to the cost-effectiveness of TBI rehabilitation programs, however, is unclear. Cope and Hall's findings [38] of substantial savings with patients admitted a month or less after injury may be explained by the superior skills of treatment teams experienced with severe head trauma compared with treatment organizations without such experience, rather than timing, per se. Furthermore, certain types of rehabilitative interventions appear to be effective even with a great delay after injury. Eames and Wood [56] admitted 30 chronic, severe TBI patients to a strict behavioral modification program an average of 4 years after injury. Before admission, these patients were either candidates for institutionalization or were actually in psychiatric institutions. There is little doubt that, by ordinary standards, these patients had plateaued and would not be considered candidates for further rehabilitation. The great majority (24 of 30) were placed in less restrictive living arrangements after discharge and remained in these improved settings for at least 18 months.

In the related field of stroke rehabilitation, recent research has found that later referrals tend to be more severe than earlier ones and that time since onset has only a very minor effect on outcomes when other factors are controlled for [57,58]. Similarly in TBI, there are a number of powerful predictors of rehabilitation outcomes; timing, per se, will probably prove useful only in conjunction with other factors.

Intensity of Rehabilitative Treatment

One encounters the belief that more therapy is always better than less. Families pressure rehabilitation staff to provide as much therapy as possible. Current standards of practice in specialized brain injury rehabilitation programs in the United States favor weeks to months of intensive, multidisciplinary therapy. But is there evidence that such intensive efforts are necessary?

A contemporary study by Fryer and Haffey [33] compared community reintegration outcomes of a 10-week outpatient cognitive retraining program with those of a 9-month residential treatment program for severely brain-injured persons after acute medical rehabilitation. None of the outpatients with moderately severe psychosocial disability (a score of 31 or greater on a psychosocial disability scale) achieved acceptable community reintegration, whereas 9 of 14 residents of the more intense residential treatment program attained "good" or "fair" community reintegration. Intense long-term treatment may then be necessary for many severely brain-injured persons to return to life in the community, but the authors thought that intensity was not the primary factor involved. The residential program also provided a more consistent learning environment than the outpatient program and aimed at providing cognitive orthoses rather than increasing cognitive function, per se.

There is also evidence that relatively inexpensive day treatment programs can be helpful. Cole et al [59] developed a community day treatment or activity program, housed in a local church, for chronic, severely brain-injured patients. Patients were admitted a mean of 25.7 months after injury and stayed in the program for a number of months. About half (47%) improved in function. Cost averaged only $3 per hour in direct expenses for labor and supplies per brain-injured "student" over the course of the program.

It is known that the total time spent in practice is highly related to the amount of task learning. But as time in a trial increases, fatigue, inattention, and diminishing motivation begin to restrict incremental gains. Many factors besides sheer time are important, including the person's level of environmental responsivity, training type, consistency of training across settings, and distribution of reinforcement. A recent study in a general rehabilitation hospital unit found that a government regulation that required indiscriminate increases in the intensity of PT and OT to a minimum of three hours per day led to no improvements in patient function, though the increase in therapy cost a great deal [60]. There is widespread agreement that younger, alert TBI survivors who are past the period of medical instability following the injury can benefit from more than three hours per day of therapy. But how much rehabilitation is optimal? Some brain injury rehabilitation facilities give 3 to 4 hours per day to patients, whereas others give 7 to 14 hours of therapy daily. Research to determine the optimal dose of rehabilitation could save millions of dollars.

Rehabilitation in a Hospital versus Skilled Nursing Facility

In the past, comprehensive intensive rehabilitation programs were available only in hospital-based facilities, and skilled nursing facilities (SNFs) typically offered only the services of a few part-time therapists. This has changed in the last few years. Comprehensive, intensive categorical brain injury programs can now be found in facilities operating on an SNF license.

Patients with medical complications requiring intensive daily management by a physician and an acute care nurse need to be treated in a hospital, and many TBI patients have such complications [61]. However, medical problems frequently recede within a few weeks after the injury, and the strictly medical needs of most TBI patients can easily be met in an SNF if certain conditions are met. Patients must be strictly screened for medical conditions that the nursing facility cannot safely handle. The nurses, doctors, and therapists in the SNF must have experience with the problems faced by the brain-injured individuals. Patient needs for a coordinated rehabilitative program do not differ across various settings.

Brain-injured patients, even ventilator-dependent ones, are increasingly being rehabilitated in nonhospital settings. One reason for this is that nursing facilities can easily be tailored to the needs of brain injury rehabilitation and can avoid paying for overhead unrelated to the needs of most TBI rehabilitation patients (e.g., the expensive medical hardware, surgical facilities, daily care by a physician, bedside oxygen, code blue teams; financial losses in the emergency room, pediatrics, or other hospital departments.) However, there are no savings in therapy staffing, because current quality standards require an SNF rehabilitation program to be staffed like an acute hospital program. Data from the New Medico Head Injury System indicate that savings of between $50 and $100 per day may be realized in SNF rehabilitation for appropriate TBI patients.

Implications of Social and Cognitive Disablement

The primary long-term disablers for TBI survivors are most frequently social-behavioral and cognitive rather than physical [62]. However, brain-injured persons are still placed in rehabilitation programs that focus most therapeutic efforts on physical disabilities and undertreat cognitive and social behavioral disabilities. Financial incentives encourage such misallocation of efforts. The medical insurance system in this country is designed to pay for medical treatment of physical impairments. Reimbursement for the cognitive and behavioral intervention in brain injury rehabilitation programs may be denied because these treatments smack of mental health or educational treatments, which are excluded by policies. The bias of insurance policies toward coverage of hospital expenses can be a problem because community-based programs can provide a more appropriate learning environment for community reintegration. These practices make no sense in brain injury rehabilitation and cannot be justified on the basis of cost effectiveness.

Another consequence of the cognitive nature of disability produced by TBI is the need for a consistent approach to rehabilitative training across treatment settings and personnel. It makes little sense for an occupational therapist to train a person to be independent in dressing or feeding in the activities of daily living room but allow the same patient to demand to be dressed and fed by nurses. Payment on a per diem rather than a fee-for-service basis could allow the rehabilitation team to distribute resources as needed to maximize patient functioning, thus encouraging greater cost-effectiveness. Mechanisms to ensure adequate staffing or treatment intensity and of monitoring patient response to treatment need to accompany per diem reimbursement.

A final implication of social-cognitive disablement is that the outcomes of TBI rehabilitation cannot be adequately measured merely by functional independence in self-care and mobility, the mainstays of physical rehabilitation programs. Social behavior, communicative functioning, and the real-world behaviors most affected by cognitive problems need to be measured [49].

Criteria for Rehabilitation Effectiveness

Cost-effectiveness is meaningless if effectiveness is not defined. Many of the complex and subtle problems in measurement of rehabilitation outcomes disappear when one takes the perspective of society, which pays for rehabilitation and which rehabilitation is supposed to serve, rather than the perspective of clinical professionals. Patients and families typically expect a major improvement in patient functioning as a consequence of rehabilitation. Insurance policies cover rehabilitation when parties to the insurance negotiation believe that rehabilitation is a substantial benefit that reduces long-term costs (e.g., attendant costs, rehospitalization costs). Rehabilitation marketing personnel sell rehabilitation by holding out the promise of substantial improvement in patient functioning and reduced long-term costs to all. In sum, society expects a robust effect of rehabilitation, and robust effects are much easier to measure than subtle ones. A great deal of useful cost-effectiveness research can proceed using fairly simple measurement tools.

There is widespread agreement that rehabilitation is effective if it causes improved functioning in practical activities of everyday life. Improvement in an impairment or artificial clinical task alone (e.g., improved range of motion, breath control, or a cognitive training task) does not justify rehabilitation if it does not lead to improvement in performance in practical ability. Neuropsychological tests, for instance, commonly lack ecological validity [63]. Improvement on such test scores is generally a poor basis on which to justify continued rehabilitation. Furthermore, even actual improvement in behavior or skill is pointless if the skill is not likely to be used or useful in the living situation of the person after discharge from rehabilitation. Substantial money might be saved by developing systems to ensure funding only when patients respond to treatment with real functional gains that are likely to be generalized to life after discharge.

Both in research and in clinical practice there is a tendency to define a set of rehabilitative goals that are common for all brain-injured individuals. In a typical inpatient rehabilitation unit, all brain-injured patients may be given a fairly standard set of therapies (PT, OT, speech, psychology, nursing, etc.). While the patient may have disabilities of the type treated by each of these professions, only one or two of these disabilities may in fact pose a critical barrier to discharge to a less restrictive living arrangement or a more productive role in life for the individual served [64]. The critical barrier may lie in the social or physical environment rather than in the disabled person. Rehabilitative efforts need to be prioritized to ensure that the greatest effort is devoted to the greatest barrier to improved outcomes.

Alternative Means to Ultimate Ends

Hundreds of cost-benefit and cost-effectiveness studies in health care have been conducted in the last two decades. Consideration of alternatives to existing or conventional programs and practices has been one of the main contributions of the more useful studies. Conversely, studies that considered only a narrow range of costs, benefits, or alternatives have more frequently been sterile or misleading. Cost-benefit and cost-effectiveness studies need to consider *all* relevant costs, benefits, and alternatives [65].

For instance, one might criticize the tendency to consider rehabilitation solely in terms of improved patient functioning exclusive of a frequently effective alternative, namely, modification of the social or physical environment. It may be far cheaper to modify a person's house to make it simpler to get around than to train the person to the point of total independence. Reminder systems may be much less expensive than months of memory training. In other cases, it may be much more practical to buy a microwave oven and train the person to turn it on than to train to total independence in cooking. Training the family to understand may in some cases be much more effective and less expensive than training the patient to speak and think more clearly. In general, flexibility of means is essential to maximizing cost-effectiveness.

Community Reintegration and Long-Term Support

The current system of care for survivors of severe brain trauma is no system at all. For some persons, no funding is available for rehabilitation. For others, funding provides incentives for continuation of rehabilitation far beyond the point where any real benefit is likely. Many survivors of TBI fall into a gap between acute medical rehabilitation and vocational rehabilitation; their functional level is too high for continuation of medical rehabilitation but too low for return to competitive employment. Funding for the community reintegration programs these patients need is scant and inconsistent. Many TBI patients are left to the care of families who suffer extraordinary stress in their attempts to cope [62]. Frequently, no insurance or governmental funding is available to help until a catastrophic event leads to rehospitalization or placement in a long-term care institution.

There are indications that the current non-system of care for brain injury survivors relies too much on institutional treatment. In related fields such as mental health, rigorous studies have shown that non-institutional, community support programs can be cost-effective compared to the usual non-system of follow-up care after discharge from psychiatric institutions [66]. Logically, savings should be possible by developing non-institutional systems for community reintegration and long-term support of brain-injured persons [67]. Such services must, however, target their interventions at the primary reasons for rehospitalization and high support costs if they are to demonstrate cost-benefits.

A central problem is that, for most patients at present, no one is responsible for an optimal or even rationally defensible balance between short-term rehabilitation and long-run support services. There is a tradeoff between expenditures for rehabilitation and long-term support of brain-injured persons and their families. If too much money is spent on one, not enough will be left for the other. Development of systems in which someone is responsible for allocating resources between rehabilitation and long-term support is needed (e.g., case management systems for catastrophic illness [68]). Such systems have the potential to be much more cost effective in both human and financial terms than the current nonsystem. Research on methods of improving long-term support of brain injury survivors and avoiding rehospitalization, institutionalization, and other untoward outcomes is a priority.

SUMMARY AND CONCLUSIONS

The costs of brain injury are larger than previously reported. Nationwide expenditures for medical care of TBI are probably between $1.9 and $2.8 billion annually in 1986 dollars. The indirect costs of lost wages are much larger: about $25.9 to $34.4 billion annually. The total annual cost of TBI would then be about $28 to $37 billion. The costs of brain injury appear to be increasing. They are not likely to diminish without major efforts and new policies aimed at prevention, improved medical care, more effective rehabilitation and long-term support, and cost control.

The key question is what interventions have the greatest impact on TBI costs. Decision making in TBI is hampered by a shortage of studies giving direct evidence of the cost-effectiveness and cost-benefits of interventions. The absence of such studies increases the likelihood of massive misallocation of resources and continuation of needless suffering. The magnitude of the costs of brain injury justifies a much larger number of studies with control groups or reliable baselines. Fortunately, methods of experimental design, outcome measurement, and research strategy relevant to cost-effectiveness and cost-benefit analysis, have improved in recent years [26,69].

Although direct study of cost-effectiveness and cost-benefits is needed, the number of combinations of treatments and policies, patient types, and outcome considerations is too great for rigorous studies of all treatment and policy alternatives ever to be completed. Decision makers need to make use of the information that already exists regarding more and less effective treatments and policies. We will always have to rely on reason to bridge voids in data.

ACKNOWLEDGMENT

Financial support for preparation of this work was provided by The New Medico Head Injury System.

REFERENCES

1. Anderson DW, McLaurin RL, eds. Report on the National Head and Spinal Cord Injury Survey. National Institute of Neurological and Communicative Disorders and Stroke. J Neurosurg 1980;53(Suppl).
2. Grabow JD, Offord KP, Rieder ME. The cost of head trauma in Olmsted County, Minnesota, 1970–74. Am J Pub Health, 1984:710–12.
3. Kalsbeek WD, McLaurin RL, Harris BS, Miller JD. The National Head and Spinal Cord Injury Survey: Major findings. J Neurosurg 1980;53(Suppl):S19–S31.
4. National Center for Health Statistics. Acute conditions. Incidence and associated disability, United States, July 1974–June 1975. Vital and Health Statistics, Series 10, No. 114. DHEW Publ No.(HRA)77-1541. Washington, DC: U.S. Government Printing Office, 1977.
5. Kraus JF. Epidemiology of head injury. In: Cooper PR, ed. Head injury. 2nd ed. Baltimore: Williams & Wilkins, 1987.
6. Annegers JF, Grabow JD, Kurland LT, Laws ER Jr. The incidence, causes, and secular trends of head trauma in Olmsted County, Minnesota, 1935-1974. Neurology 1980;30:912–19.
7. Field JH. Epidemiology of head injuries in England and Wales. London: Department of Health and Social Security, Her Majesty's Stationcry Office, 1976.
8. Jennett B. Scale and scope of the problem. In: Rosenthal M, Griffith ER, Bond MR, and Miller JD, eds. Rehabilitation of the head injured adult. Philadelphia: F.A. Davis, 1983;3–8.
9. Committee on Trauma Research, Commission on Life Sciences, National Research Council, and the Institute of Medicine, National Academy of Sciences. Injury in America. Washington, DC: National Academy Press, 1985.
10. Kraus JF, Black MA, Hessol N, Ley P, Rokaw W, Sullivan C, Bowers S, Knowlton

S, Marshall L. The incidence of acute brain injury and serious impairment in a defined population. Am J Epidemiol 1984;119:186–201.

11. Jane J, Rimel R, Poberskin L, Tyson G, Steward O, Genarelli T. Outcome and pathology of head injury. In: Grossman R, Gildenberg P, eds. Head injury: Basic and clinical aspects. New York: Raven, 1982;229–37.

12. Wagner K. Brain injury: A prospective outcome study. Paper presented at the Fifth Annual Traumatic Head Injury Conference. Braintree, MA, October 17–19, 1984.

13. Dresser M, Meirowsky AM, Weiss GH, McNeel ML, Simon GA, Caveness WF. Gainful employment following head injury. Arch Neurol 1973;29:111–16.

14. Gilchrist E, Wilkinsen M. Some factors determining prognosis in young people with severe head injuries. Arch Neurol 1979;36:355–59.

15. Brennan M. Resumption of work following discharge from hospital. Irish Med J 1981;74:5–7.

16. Lewin W, Marshall TFDC, Roberts AH. Long-term outcome after severe head injury. Br Med J 15 Dec 1979;1533–38.

17. Oddy M, Humphrey M. Social recovery during the year following severe head injury. J Neurol Neurosurg Psychiatry 1980;43:798–802.

18. Brooks DN, McKinlay W, Symington C, Beattie A, Campsie L. Return to work within the first seven years of severe head injury. Brain injury 1987;1:5–19.

19. Prigatano GP, Klonoff PS, Bailey I. Psychosocial adjustment associated with traumatic brain injury: Statistics BNI neurorehabilitation must beat. BNI Quarterly 1987;3(1):10–17.

20. Jacobs HE: Los Angeles head injury survey: Procedures and initial findings. Arch Phys Med Rehabil 1988;69:425–31.

21. Rice DP. Estimating the cost of illness. US DHEW, PHS Pub. 947-6, Health Economics Series No 6, Washington, DC: US Government Publishing Office, 1966.

22. Committee on Trauma Research, Commission on Life Sciences, National Research Council and the Institute of Medicine. Injury in America. Washington,DC: National Academy Press, 1985.

23. Robertson LS. Injuries. Causes, control strategies, and public policy. Lexington, MA: DC Heath, 1983.

24. Baker SP, O'Neill B, Karpf RS. The injury fact book. Lexington, MA: DC Heath, 1984.

25. McSwain NE, Petrucelli E. Medical consequences of motorcycle helmet nonusage. J Trauma 1984;24:233–36.

26. Warner KE, Luce BR. Cost-benefit and cost-effectiveness analysis in health care. Ann Arbor, MI: Health Administration Press, 1982.

27. Henry WR, Haynes WE. Managerial economics. 4th ed. Dallas, TX: Business Publications, 1978.

28. Mendelow AD, Campbell DA, Jeffrey RR, Miller JD, Hessett C, Bryden J, Jennett B. Admission after mild head injury: Benefits and costs. Br Med J; Nov 27, 1982:1285–87.

29. Reiner DS, Hurd R, Smith K, Kaminski DL. Selective peritoneal lavage in the management of comatose blunt trauma patients. J Trauma 1986;26:255–59.

30. Bartkowski HM, Lovely MP. Prognosis in coma and the persistent vegetative state. J Head Trauma Rehabil 1986;1:1–5.

31. Berrol S. Evolution and the persistent vegetative state. J Head Trauma Rehabil 1986;1:7–13.

32. Jennett B. Resource allocation for the severely brain damaged. Arch Neurol 1976;33:595–97.
33. Fryer LJ, Haffey WJ. Cognitive rehabilitation and community readaptation: outcomes from two program models. J Head Trauma Rehabil 1987;2(3):51–63.
34. Giannotta SL, Weiner JM, Karnaze D. Prognosis and outcome in severe head injury. In: Cooper PR, ed. Head injury. 2nd ed. Baltimore: Williams & Wilkins, 1987;464–87.
35. Berrol S. Considerations for managment of persistent vegetative state. Arch Phys Med Rehabil 1986;67:283–85.
36. National Association of Rehabilitation Facilities, Coopers and Lybrand. Prospective payment study. NARF Medex survey. Data analysis. Washington, DC: National Association of Rehabilitation Facilities, February 5, 1985.
37. Hosek S, Kane R, Carney M, Hartman J, Reboussin D, Serrato C, Melvin J. Charges and outcomes for rehabilitative care: Implications for the prospective payment system. Santa Monica, CA: Rand Corporation, 1986.
38. Cope DN, Hall K. Head injury rehabilitation: benefit of early intervention. Arch Phys Med Rehabil 1982;63:433–37.
39. Aronow HU. Rehabilitation effectiveness with severe brain injury. J Head Injury Rehabil 1987;2(3):24–36.
40. Carey RG, Posavac EJ, Seibert JH. Who makes the most progress in inpatient rehabilitation? An analysis of functional gain. Arch Phys Med Rehabil 1988;69:337–43.
41. Harasymiw SJ, Albrecht GL. Admission and discharge indicators as aids in optimizing comprehensive rehabilitation services. Scand J Rehabil Med 1979;11:123–38.
42. Johnston MV, Miller LS. Efficiency of inpatient rehabilitation: Measurement by improvement per dollar. Arch Phys Med Rehabil 1986;67:632.
43. Johnston MV, Keith RA. Cost-benefits of medical rehabilitation: Review and critique. Arch Phys Med Rehabil 1983;64:147–54.
44. Hall KM, Cope DN. The current status of head injury rehabilitation. In: Miner ME, Wagner KA, eds. Neurotrauma: Treatment, rehabilitation, and related issues. No. 1. Boston: Butterworths, 1986;223–32.
45. Berkowitz M. Bureau of Economic Research. Analysis of costs and benefits in rehabilitation: Final report. New Brunswick, NJ: Rutgers University, 1985.
46. Fuhrer MJ. Medical rehabilitation research: Distortions, deflections and detractions. Arch Phys Med Rehabil 1982;63:49–54.
47. Fuhrer MJ. Evaluating a funding agency's performance: A rehabilitation researcher's perspective. Arch Phys Med Rehabil 1982;63:190–91.
48. World Health Organization. International classification of impairments, disabilities and handicaps. Geneva: World Health Organization, 1980.
49. Haffey WJ, Johnston MV. An information system to assess the effectiveness of brain injury rehabilitation. In: Wood R, Eames P, eds. Models of brain injury rehabilitation. London: Chapman & Hall. In press.
50. Caplan B. Neuropsychology in rehabilitation. Arch Phys Med Rehabil 1982;63:362–66.
51. Cope DN. Traumatic closed head injury: Status of rehabilitation treatment. Semin Neurol 1985;5:212–18.
52. Ben-Yishay Y, Diller L. Cognitive remediation. In: Rosenthal M, Griffith ER, Bond MR, Miller JD, eds. Rehabilitation of the head injured adult. Philadelphia: Davis, 1983;367–80.

53. Matsun JL, McCartney JR, eds. Handbook of behavior modification with the mentally retarded. New York: Plenum, 1981.

54. Schacter DL, Glisky EL. Memory remediation: restoration, alleviation, and the acquisition of domain-specific knowledge. In: Uzzell BP, Gross Y, eds. Clinical neuropsychology of intervention. Boston: Martinus Nijhoff, 1986;257–82.

55. Lord JP, Hall K. Neuromuscular reeducation versus traditional programs for stroke rehabilitation. Arch Phys Med Rehabil 1986;67:88–91.

56. Eames P, Wood R. Rehabilitation after severe brain injury: a follow-up study of a behavior modification approach. J Neurol Neurosurg Psychiatry 1985;48:613–19.

57. Johnston MV, Keister M. Early rehabilitation for stroke patients: a new look. Arch Phys Med Rehabil 1984;65:437–41.

58. Novack TA, Satterfield WT, Connor M. Stroke onset and rehabilitation: time lag as a factor in treatment outcome. Arch Phys Med Rehabil 1984;65:316–19.

59. Cole JR, Cope DN, Cervelli L. Rehabilitation of the severely brain injured patient: A community-based, low-cost model program. Arch Phys Med Rehabil 1985;66:38–40.

60. Johnston MV, Miller LS. Cost-effectiveness of the Medicare three-hour regulation. Arch Phys Med Rehabil 1986;67:581–85.

61. Miller LS, Johnston MV. Necessary medical care for inpatient rehabilitation. Arch Phys Med Rehabil 1986;67:612.

62. Brooks N. Closed head injury: Psychological, social, and family consequences. Oxford: Oxford University Press, 1984.

63. Hart T, Hayden ME. The ecological validity of neuropsychological assessment and remediation. In: Uzzell BP, Gross Y, eds. Clinical neuropsychology of intervention. Boston: Martinus Nijhoff, 1986:21–50.

64. Haffey WJ, Johnston MJ. A functional assessment system for real world rehabilitation outcomes. In: Tupper D, Cicerone K, eds. The neuropsychology of everyday life. Boston: Martinus Nijhoff. In press.

65. Office of Technology Assessment, Congress of the United States. Assessing the efficacy and safety of medical technologies. Washington, DC: U.S. Government Printing Office, 1978.

66. Weisbrud BA, Test MA, Stein LI. Alternative to mental hospital treatment. II. Economic benefit-cost analysis. Arch Gen Psychiatry 37;1980:392–97.

67. Johnston MV, Cervelli L. Systematic care for persons with head injury. In: Bachy-Rita P, ed. Traumatic brain injury. NY: Demos. In press.

68. Henderson MG, Wallack SS. Evaluating case management for catastrophic illness. Business Health, January 1987:7–11.

69. Johnston MV. Cost-benefit methodologies in rehabilitation. In: Fuhrer MJ, ed. Rehabilitation outcomes: Analysis and measurement. Baltimore: Brookes, 1987;99–114.

Chapter 15

Neurotrauma and Medical Malpractice

Robert W. Rand

The risk of medical malpractice is greatest when the injured person first enters the emergency treatment facility. At the University of California at Los Angeles (UCLA) Hospital Trauma Center, we have had three cases of medical malpractice that will be used here to illustrate the Tort of Negligence. Each case involved trauma victims who were clearly inappropriately managed, and settlements were made in order to prevent higher awards that surely would have been given in a California Superior Court jury trial. The information is no longer confidential because each case against the Regents of the University of California has been terminated.

CASE 1

A 19-year-old man, while performing pulling weight exercises in the gym of his apartment building, began having symptoms of nausea, shortness of breath, pain in the abdomen, numbness in the lower extremities, and inability to walk. He arrived at the UCLA Trauma Center via ambulance approximately 29 minutes after the onset of symptoms. He was seen by a surgical intern and a psychiatric resident who, after observing him, made a diagnosis of "conversion hysteria." They provided no neurologic work-up, nor did they refer the patient to the UCLA neurosurgical or neurological services, which were readily available. The patient was discharged and told to see a psychiatrist or go to Camarillo State Hospital for the mentally ill. After discharge from the UCLA Trauma Center his symptoms increased. Following the physicians' instructions, he was taken to a psychiatric counseling center and from there to another hospital where he was operated upon for decompression of the thoracic spinal cord some days after the onset of symptoms. Because of the delay in neurological work-up and the consequent delay in surgical intervention to remove the ruptured thoracic disk and bleeding into the spinal cord, the patient is now paraplegic.

In the decision to recommend settlement, the UCLA Medical Risk Management Committee was influenced by the following:

1. The physician who actually made the diagnosis was a surgical intern, and it was his first week of surgery service at the UCLA Trauma Center. The psychiatric consult was given by a resident whose personnel file contained several letters questioning his competency to practice medicine.
2. The emergency center records on the patient were scant, with no background history, no description of the time or manner of onset of symptoms, and only a superficial preliminary examination.
3. No neurological or neurosurgical consultation was called at any time.
4. The plaintiff's attorney intended to provide testimony from experts in emergency room procedures indicating that the organizational and supervisional aspects of the UCLA Trauma Center were entirely insufficient. It seemed probable that there was little that could be said in defense of the care rendered.
5. Expert neurosurgical testimony would have produced evidence at trial that bleeding into the spinal cord was progressive and that prompt intervention would have left the patient no worse than ambulatory with crutches.

The verdict potential at trial could have been in the multimillion dollar range. The case had definite hazards, and the UCLA attorneys felt justified in making the $500,000 settlement.

CASE 2

A 41-year-old woman was involved in a rather serious auto accident and taken via ambulance to the UCLA Trauma Center. The two primary physicians who saw her were a surgical resident and a psychiatric resident. In the course of the examination various roentgenograms were obtained and read as negative. She was kept in the facility from approximately 10 A.M. until 8 P.M., at which time she was discharged with the following diagnoses: (1) loss of left upper incisor; (2) small laceration of the dorsum of the right foot; (3) multiple soft tissue contusions; (4) conversion hysteria.

The patient returned the following morning after spending the night immobilized on a makeshift stretcher. She was seen in the UCLA Neuropsychiatric Institute Emergency Room, where her admission to the UCLA Neurosurgery Unit was arranged. The final diagnosis was transverse myelopathy at C-7, which was almost complete and which was secondary to hyperextension of the neck. She was discharged to Rancho Los Amigos Rehabilitation Hospital. The patient can now walk with the aid of a walker but has only partial control of her bladder and requires medication for elimination.

The reasons for settlement were:

1. The diagnostic error was quite serious. There was clear evidence in the patient's chart that the first neurological examination in the UCLA Trauma Center must have been abnormal, and a neurological or a neurosurgical consult should have been obtained.
2. The recorded history in the patient's chart concerning the makeshift stretcher and an attempt to admit her to psychiatry would produce a very adverse reaction in any sympathetic listener, such as a member of a California jury.
3. When the UCLA Trauma Center log was subpoenaed it was found that the times of admission and discharge of the patient had been erased and entries had been changed.
4. The only UCLA hospital defense in this case would be that premature discharge from the Trauma Center did not influence the subsequent outcome of the patient's neurological difficulty, due to the nonsurgical nature of the spinal cord syndrome. The UCLA defense attorneys could not find expert physicians to agree to testify to this.

Had this case gone to trial it would have been difficult to defend the UCLA Medical Risk Management Committee, and the verdict at trial would probably have been in the million dollar range. The case was settled out of court for $400,000.

CASE 3

A young man was admitted to the UCLA Trauma Center complaining of having been struck on the head by a tire iron. The emergency record reflects a thorough and appropriate physical examination of the scalp wound. Digital and visual exploration were performed and did not reveal a depressed skull fracture. However, no skull roentgenograms were taken at that time, nor was a CT scan performed. Afterward, the patient continued to have severe headaches. On day 4 postinjury, meningismus developed and he was hospitalized. He was found to have a depressed skull fracture, which was operated upon and elevated eight days after injury.

The patient had received an adequately thorough physical assessment. The care of his soft tissue wound was appropriate. In those areas the care he received met or exceeded the general standard of care in teaching hospitals.

The way in which the care and treatment of this patient may not have met these standards is that no skull roentgenogram or CT scan was taken. Had such studies been done, the depressed skull fracture would have been detected. It might be argued that a thorough physical examination ought to have detected the skull fracture. But that is not necessarily true because the galea of the scalp may be intact in such wounds, and the interposed hematoma may make it impossible to feel the depressed fracture of the skull. The patient signed the usual consent form for patients seen in the UCLA Trauma Center, but there is no indication that the physician discussed with him whether a skull roentgenogram or CT scan was indicated. That is, there is no indication that the doctor gave his patient the opportunity to "request" a skull roentgenogram or brain image.

The position of UCLA in this case is relatively weak, and settlement was recommended. In failing to obtain a skull roentgenogram or CT scan on this patient the physician was following a set of "high-yield criteria" for indication for skull radiography. His decision not to order a skull roentgenogram based on these criteria is probably defensible from a purely professional point of view, because these criteria had been described in the medical literature and had been advocated by governmental agencies as the way to reduce the cost of emergency care without reducing its quality. However, because of the rather dramatic nature of the patient's case, and particularly the mechanism of the skull injury by a tire iron, the hospital's position would be weak in a court of law before a jury.

As a result of this case and similar cases that have occurred in other institutions in the Los Angeles community, most emergency physicians are now aware that the use of the so-called high-yield criteria will cause physicians to miss small depressed skull fractures in certain patients whose mechanism of injury is similar to a ball peen hammer. This information has been repeatedly disseminated to UCLA resident physicians, and the necessity of skull radiography in such injuries has become axiomatic. Even better than skull roentgenograms, and equally able to detect skull fractures, especially at the skull base, is the CT scan using the CT bone window settings. In addition, brain edema and small brain hemorrhages can be identified and treated. Furthermore, x-ray dosage is less with CT than with a complete set of skull roentgenograms.

This case was settled for $3,500.

TORT OF NEGLIGENCE

The Tort of Negligence would be applicable to each of these cases. The earliest appearance of the concept of negligence was in the liability of persons considered competent in selected public activities [1]. A surgeon is regarded as one in whom public confidence might be placed and who therefore assumes an obligation to give proper surgical care. Initially, negligence concerned positive acts rather than omissions. In the early nineteenth century, negligence was recognized as a separate tort liability. Today, separate problems and principles of tort law apply to both action and inaction, and questions of legal policy arise in negligence cases.

Liability founded upon negligence requires more than conduct. The traditional formula for the elements of the Tort of Negligence necessary to a Cause of Action are: a duty requiring the action to conform to a certain standard of conduct established for protection against unreasonable risks, and a failure on the defendant's part to conform to this reasonable standard.

Although both these elements are required to define negligence, the term is frequently applied to the latter alone because the former is assumed. The close causal connection between a defendant's conduct and an injury is known as legal or proximate cause. Clearly the three cases cited do fulfill the criteria of medical negligence, that is, the omission of a duty that resulted in a proximate cause of damage to the patients.

STATUTE OF LIMITATIONS

In the past the statute of limitations began to run at the time of injury. Frequently, in cases of medical malpractice the statutes ran out before patients discovered that they had suffered any injury. That injustice led to the adoption of legal devices to circumvent the rule. Thus, the statute of limitations begins either when a patient discovers the injury or when a prudent person should have discovered the injury. Fraudulent concealment of damage clearly stops the running of the statute of limitations. Failure to discover or remove foreign objects left in the plaintiff's body is held to be "continuing negligence" for which there is no statute of limitations.

BASIS OF NEGLIGENCE

The real basis of negligence is behavior that should be recognized as involving unreasonable danger to others. However, the burden is on the plaintiff from the onset to establish unreasonable risk. Negligent conduct is determined by balancing the risk and the probability of harm. Conduct that would be proper under some circumstances becomes negligent under others.

The courts have created "the reasonable man of ordinary prudence." However, the physician is actually required to do what an ideal individual would be supposed to do in this profession. Negligence is a failure to do what "the reasonable man" would do under similar circumstances. In medicine, what was excusable ignorance yesterday becomes negligent ignorance today. However, juries are composed of lay persons normally incompetent to pass judgment on questions of medical science or technique. Therefore, in the majority of malpractice cases there can be no finding of negligence in the absence of expert testimony. The summation of these legal rules is that the standard of conduct simply becomes one of "good medical practice" that is customary and usual in the professional community. Because the standard is a community standard, evidence of the usual and customary conduct of others under similar circumstances is normally relevant and admissible as an indication of what the community regards as proper, combined with the judgment as to risks and precautions. Omission of customary conduct may in itself be a cause for negligence, especially where it is known that others may rely on such customary conduct.

SPORTS INJURIES

In 1972, Norrell discussed the neurosurgeon's responsibility in the prevention of sports injuries [2]. This concept opened a new liability for neurosurgeons because an ever-increasing number of students and professionals are involved in increasingly violent physical sports. Therefore, in addition to the legal concepts of contributory negligence and the assumption of risks, there has emerged the concept of shared negligence. The question often is: Does the "team neurosurgeon" have a shared negligence with an athlete if the neurosurgeon knew or should have known that a particular risk existed for an athlete under his or her care? Norrell concluded that injuries to the nervous system are not uncommon accompaniments of sports and the neurosurgeon's role should extend beyond the immediate recognition and treatment of sports injuries to the nervous system. The neurosurgeon must not only be prepared to evaluate the injured player but also to give a reasonable assessment of the severity of the injury as related to future sports participation. The neurosurgeon must not allow the patient to return to the sport before he or she has recovered, and likewise should not withhold participation for an unduly long time. This has become a difficult burden and conduct potentially carrying high liability.

Furthermore, Norrell imposes upon the neurosurgeon the responsibility of educating team physicians, coaches, and trainers because neurosurgeons cannot be at every sports event. The medical malpractice liability of a team neurosurgeon will increase substantially as the concept of prevention of injuries is accepted by the courts. Thus, a neurosurgeon should weigh carefully the professional benefit against the risks of a malpractice action when accepting such an assignment as team neurosurgeon. In the case of college or professional sports, the cost of such malpractice should be borne by the institution or team rather than the neurosurgeon.

SETTLEMENT

In 1985 Fager published a retrospective review of 300 cases of alleged or potential liability to evaluate the highest risk to neurosurgeons [3]. The single largest group of neurosurgical malpractice cases (45%) was related to spinal surgery, with cerebral and spinal trauma accounting for another 18%. Of these 300 cases, 46% had some merit in favor of the plaintiff whereas the remainder had no merit. Mistakes and accidents will always be with us, but most serious liability should be preventable provided one has an understanding of the legal elements of the Tort of Negligence. It is difficult to escape the conclusion that juries consider serious neurological disability compensable regardless of fault, believing that physicians and hospitals are insured. The most frequently mentioned solution is no-fault or maloccurrence insurance. As my father, Carl W. Rand, a neurosurgeon trained by Dr. Harvey Cushing used to say, "a malpractice trial is no truth-telling contest." There have also been suggestions that jury trials should be eliminated altogether and replaced by boards of arbitration.

REFERENCES

1. Negligence "Standard of Conduct." In: Prosser and Keeton on the law of torts. 5th ed. St. Paul, MN: West Publishing Co., 1984;160–262;451–98.
2. Norrel H. The neurosurgeon's responsibility in the prevention of sports injuries. In: Tindall G, Wilkins R, Keener E, Meyer G, eds. Clinical neurosurgery. Baltimore: Williams & Wilkins, 1971;208–19.
3. Fager C. Professional liability and potential liability. Neurosurgery 1985;16:866–72.

Chapter 16

Trends in Brain Injury Rehabilitation and Research: The Past Ten Years and Future Challenges

Mitchell Rosenthal

The past decade has seen an enormous growth of interest in rehabilitation after traumatic brain injury. Published research has burgeoned and brain injury rehabilitation facilities have proliferated, and the medical community, social agencies, and legislative systems now acknowledge that brain injury is a unique diagnostic entity requiring a specialized approach to management.

Research has led to a better understanding of the course of recovery from brain injury; the nature of long-term residual neurobehavioral disorders after minor, moderate, and severe brain injury; the use of neuropsychological assessment techniques to evaluate progress, plan interventions, and predict outcome; the development and widespread use of cognitive and behavioral rehabilitation techniques to improve long-term outcome; and the inclusion of the family in the rehabilitation process and the examination of the effects of traumatic brain injury on them [1]. These are but a few of the major advances in knowledge and rehabilitation that have occurred. Yet there have been few well-controlled research studies documenting the scientific reliability and validity of rehabilitation interventions.

MEDICAL MANAGEMENT

Within the broad areas of acute and rehabilitative management, a number of major advances can be delineated. First, a number of epidemiologic studies since 1980 have brought to light the enormous magnitude of the problem of brain injury. It is now common knowledge that: at least 500,000 brain injuries requiring admission to the hospital occur annually in the United States; at least 50,000 persons per year are left with severe residual deficits—mental, physical,

"

or both; the age group most at risk is 15 to 29 years old; males outnumber females 3 to 1; in excess of $4 billion per year is spent on medical care and lost in wages; and the extent of this so-called "silent" epidemic shows no signs of abating [2].

In the last 10 years a variety of neurodiagnostic techniques have been introduced that improve or have the potential of improving, early medical managment. These include the following: universal use of the CT scan to visualize structural lesions within the brain; use of cortical evoked potentials to assess the extent of brain dysfunction and predict outcome and occasional use of the positron emission tomography (PET) scan, which shows promise in highlighting the area of functional impairment, such as in cognitive ability. The newest technique, magnetic resonance imaging, is said to be able to visualize tiny microscopic white matter lesions that can be devastating for a brain-injured patient but cannot be seen on a CT scan [3]. It may also be useful in finding small lesions in cases of minor brain injury where normal CT scans have often been assumed to indicate lack of neuropathology.

Our ability to predict the likelihood of posttraumatic epilepsy has also improved. More judicious and selective use of anticonvulsant medication for prophylaxis has been achieved. Drugs like carbamazepine, which has a lesser effect than phenytoin on cognition, have been strongly advocated and are in use at many centers [4].

Perhaps the most significant change in medical management has been attitudinal. Neurologists and neurosurgeons recognize that rehabilitation intervention should begin very early, even in the intensive care unit. Use of the physiatrist as a consultant to neurosurgeon and in ordering treatments and therapies at an early point has likely been responsible for reducing secondary medical complications and has encouraged earlier transfer to the rehabilitation unit. Few studies, however, have documented the effectiveness of early rehabilitation.

One exception is the study by Cope and Hall [5], which retrospectively studied matched groups of brain-injured patients with coma of less than 15 days and suggested that individuals who were referred late to rehabilitation spent a much greater time in the acute hospital and at a much greater cost for total hospitalization. However, there was no difference in outcome measures when both groups were reevaluated at 2-year follow-up.

Our ability to track and predict the course of physical and neurobehavioral recovery has also improved. Instruments such as the Glasgow Outcome Scale [6], Disability Rating Scale [7], and Rancho Los Amigos Levels of Cognitive Functioning Scale [8] have proved useful in this regard. Follow-up studies performed by the Glasgow group, the Galveston group, and others have demonstrated that certain functions, like mobility, activities of daily living, and speech and language, tend to recover relatively rapidly (i.e., within the first six months), but that more complex areas of cognition and behavior have a longer recovery process (perhaps several years) [9–11]. These studies have enabled the clinician to be more comfortable in educating and counseling families as to what to expect. However, the seasoned clinician knows that in brain injury there are a thousand exceptions to every rule.

THERAPEUTIC INTERVENTION

In the area of therapeutic intervention, a number of trends have been evident. Cognitive and behavioral dysfunction have been recognized as significant to all areas of therapy; the nature of these deficits must be understood in order to provide adequate therapy to patients [12]. There has been a greater emphasis on functional, real-life activities. For example, physical therapists focus not only on transfers from wheelchair to bed and gait training, but also on community mobility skills, such as taking public transportation and driving an automobile. Occupational therapists have become concerned with activities such as money management, food shopping, and independent living skills as well as higher-level cognitive functions. Both speech therapists and occupational therapists have assumed a central role on most teams in providing intensive work on such cognitive skills as memory, organizational skills, and functional communication. The advent of computer-based augmentative communication devices has been important for many persons who are speech impaired from brain injuries. The therapeutic team has also expanded to include some newer members; the recreational therapist, case manager, special educator, and vocational specialist are often primary members of the rehabilitation team.

Neuropsychological Assessment and Treatment

Clinical neuropsychology has emerged as a critical discipline within rehabilitation. A few major contributions of the last decade include the research of Brooks [13] on cognitive function, particularly in memory; Lezak [14] on the effects of brain injury on executive function and the role of neuropsychological assessment and its effects on long-term adaptation; Levin et al [9] on the neurobehavioral sequelae of brain injury in adults and children; Bond [15] on the effects of head injury on the family; and Rimel et al [16] on the particular neuropsychological consequences of minor brain injury.

As a result of this research, we are now quite familiar with the many neurobehavioral problems that result from severe and minor brain injury. The process of neuropsychological assessment has almost gained preeminence in the evaluation of persons with brain injury, but some have seriously questioned the relevance and predictive power of many test procedures [17]. Neuropsychological assessment has, however, served as a primary means of tracking recovery, predicting outcome, planning treatment and placement, and determining future educational and vocational plans [18].

Among recent advances in clinical neuropsychology, cognitive retraining has been perhaps the most exciting and promising area of clinical investigation and research. The pioneering work of Ben-Yishay et al at New York University has spawned many cognitive retraining programs, and elements within comprehensive rehabilitation programs [19,20]. The notion that cognitive and interpersonal dysfunctions so common after brain injury can be modified through the use of a systematic methodology aimed at specific areas such as attention, visual perception, motor dexterity, or social skills has given great hope to clinicians and families of brain-injured patients. Previously, significant improvements in these areas were thought unlikely due to irreversible brain damage. The popularity of Luria's theory of functional systems [21] within the brain has also been responsible for much of the "excitement" in this area. However, there have been few well-controlled studies that definitively demonstrate that the process of cognitive retraining actually produces significant functional improvements in cognitive processes. The work of Prigatano et al [22] is one notable exception. They have demonstrated that a neuropsychologically based, 6-month rehabilitation program can improve the functional skills of brain-injured patients, as compared with a group of untreated controls, even when only modest improvements are noted on standardized neuropsychological assessment. Improvements in adaptive function and vocational capacity were found in the treatment group, even though several years had elapsed between time of injury and treatment.

The microcomputer has also had a role in cognitive retraining. In the late 1970s, Lynch [23] introduced the notion that the playing of video games by brain-injured patients could have therapeutic as well as recreational value. As society in general embraced personal computers, clinicians started to become interested in using computer programs for cognitive retraining. Gianutsos [24] and Bracey [25], among others, have designed specialized computer programs to improve deficient areas such as memory, visual perception, reaction time, and attention. Some research has demonstrated that a brain-injured person's performance on these training programs can be improved with practice, yet there has been no study demonstrating significant functional improvements in everyday aspects of cognition and living skills. One must be mindful of the accumulating data suggesting that direct retraining of skills like memory, whether through the use of memory retraining software or drill and repetition exercises, does not appear to be producing functional changes [26]. Also, the outcome studies of major cognitive rehabilitation programs such as at New York University [20] and Oklahoma-Presbyterian Hospital [22] are showing little change on neuropsychological measures, although the patients in these studies may in fact be progressing to higher functional levels. A likely explanation is that cognitive retraining programs are successful in teaching compensatory strategies, and that neuropsychological assessment techniques may not be the best methods for program evaluation.

Family Involvement

Another major trend in brain injury rehabilitation has been the inclusion of family members as active participants in the rehabilitation process. This trend may be traced to several key factors. The research of Brooks et al in Europe [27] has demonstrated that brain injury has a great impact on the entire family system. The burden of caring for a brain-injured relative is enormous, particularly if the patient has enduring behavioral or psychiatric problems. Stresses do not diminish over time; they wax and wane. Family members often have psychological difficulties of their own and need medication or psychological intervention. The second major factor has been the birth of the National Head Injury Foundation in 1980 and its proliferation as a nationwide organization of families advocating for their loved ones. Family support groups have sprung up in virtually every state and have undoubtedly been of tremendous help. From the perspective of rehabilitation, families are brought into the process very early and are often used as therapeutic agents, even when the patient is in coma. Families are given extensive education about brain injury, in groups or individually. Family counseling and family therapy are often valuable. Jacobs and Muir [28] at the UCLA Neuropsychiatric Institute are currently systematically measuring the effects of training family members as therapeutic agents for brain-injured relatives.

Behavioral Management

Another area of rehabilitation that has become a focus is the management of behavioral problems. These are varied and often quite disruptive after brain injury. Before the late 1970s, behavior problems in brain-injured patients were viewed as similar to cognitive deficits: they were a reflection of permanent brain damage and could not be changed. This thinking has changed greatly since the methods of behavior therapy have been applied successfully to many problems manifested by the brain injured. Perhaps the most well-known program based on a behavioral approach is the Kemsley Unit in Britain, whose leading exponents, Eames and Wood, have become well known in America. They have demonstrated that the use of the token economy, well established for other diagnostic populations, can have equally successful results with the brain injured [29]. Wood [30] also reported on a variety of other behavioral techniques, such as overlearning, negative reinforcement, and time-out to alter maladaptive behavior.

Even more encouraging was a study by Eames and Wood [29] demonstrating that behavior change accomplished through a token economy approach could be maintained up to one year after discharge from hospital. In severely brain-injured patients, behavioral approaches are sometimes ineffective. Thus, there has been perhaps a greater use of various medications to control behavior. Lithium has been used in very agitated patients [31]; psychostimulant medications have been used in lethargic patients [32]; and antidepressants have occasionally produced good results in depressed patients [33]. There have not yet been sufficient studies to definitely recommend any particular class of drugs. It is important to recognize that many psychotropic drugs do more harm than good in the brain injured because they can greatly alter or cloud attentional function and cognition in general [34].

Another method to improve socially inappropriate behavior has been social skills training, often in groups. Helfenstein and Wechsler [35] have suggested the use of videotape feedback of behavior in group sessions to aid patients with memory deficits in looking critically at their behavior. This was termed interpersonal process recall. It is now commonplace for most brain injury centers to use group treatment for many different disorders, such as those of language, social behavior, and vocational exploration. Prigatano, in his recent book, presents a detailed description of how to do group psychotherapy with the brain injured; he clearly believes it to be a valuable therapeutic tool [36].

Types of Rehabilitation Programs

Renewed faith in the potential for rehabilitation to improve outcome in brain-injured patients has led to a tremendous upsurge in the number and variety of programs attempting to serve the multifaceted needs of this population [37]. In 1976, only acute rehabilitation programs and nursing homes were widespread. The most universal trend has been toward the establishment of categorical brain injury units within rehabilitation facilities. Whereas brain-injured patients were previously part of mixed-diagnosis units, most large facilities that have a steady influx of brain-injured patients treat them in a geographically separate unit, often with a dedicated team of professionals who specialize in brain injury. Most clinicians, administrators, and consumers view this approach as beneficial; to date, however, no studies have found that brain-injured individuals progress faster or to a higher level in such a unit.

Another trend has been for brain injury rehabilitation programs to be located in free-standing, community-based facilities, rather than connected to a large general hospital. Often, these units are within nursing homes or psychiatric treatment facilities that have constructed new facilities on their grounds. Because third-party reimbursement constraints have shortened the length of hospitalization for all diagnostic groups, day treatment programs have emerged. In this model, a wide variety of therapeutic services are provided to the patient, often just after discharge from the acute facility. The patient attends the program five days per week, 5 to 6 hours per day and receives intensive cognitive remediation, behavior management, pre-vocational training, and the like [38].

Attempts to complete the reentry process have been aided by transitional living programs or residential facilities that emphasize the development of community living skills [39]. These facilities are not as numerous as traditional brain injury rehabilitation units, and little is known about their long-term effectiveness. This final step in community reentry is likely the hardest. The process of learning to balance a checkbook, shop at a food store, take public transportation, live with a roommate, and remember and perform many daily living routines in a timely and efficient manner requires the highest levels of cognitive integrity and behavioral control. Yet these skills will likely determine the ultimate success or failure of our rehabilitation efforts. Until these programs are commonplace and financially accessible to all brain-injured persons, other types of rehabilitation programs may have to incorporate independent living skills training into their programs.

Advocacy, Public Policy, and Brain Injury

The major advances in brain injury rehabilitation are due to a variety of factors, not the least of which has been a heightened public awareness of the problem of brain injury and massive efforts on the part of social and legislative agencies to effect change in public policy and rehabilitation practices. In this section, a brief description of the major efforts of these agencies will be described.

The National Head Injury Foundation (NHIF), started in 1980 in Framingham, Massachusetts, has come of age within the past few years. Starting out as a small group of professionals and consumers, it has expanded to encompass 25 state chapters, 350 support groups nationwide, and numerous affiliated associations. The NHIF has been largely responsible for the increase in federal funding for brain injury rehabilitation research and has played a key advocacy role that has led to the passage of seat belt laws, child restraint laws, and the development of state-supported programs for the brain-injured. NHIF, as of last year, produced an interagency agreement, signed by seven major federal agencies, that has paved the way for increased awareness and increased funding for brain injury.

The National Institute of Neurological, Communication Disorders and Stroke (as part of the National Institutes of Health) has been responsible for the vast majority of large-scale epidemiologic, acute management, animal model experimentation, and multicenter coma data bank studies that have produced a wealth of data within the past decade. One hopes that future research priorities will include a heavier emphasis on rehabilitation research, per se.

The National Institute for Handicapped Research (NIHR), now renamed The National Institute of Disability and Rehabilitation Research (NIDRR) (part of the U.S. Department of Education) came into existence in the late 1970s. At that time, they funded two major research projects in traumatic brain injury, the Santa Clara Valley Study and the New York University (NYU) Cognitive Remediation study. In a bold step in 1983, NIHR established brain injury as a priority research area and funded four brain injury and stroke rehabilitation research centers: NYU, Emory, Northwestern-Rehabilitation Institute of Chicago, and the University of Washington. This commitment of more than $2 million to brain injury research encompasses more than 45 individual research projects that show great promise in improving our understanding of the process of brain injury rehabilitation. Most recently, this agency funded five programs (Mount Sinai Hospital, New York: The Institute for Rehabilitation and Research; Santa Clara Valley Hospital; Medical College of Virginia; and Rehabilitation Institute of Detroit) to be part of a model system of service delivery and research for the traumatically brain-injured. This is quite similar to the spinal cord injury model care systems, set up in the early 1970s, which have had a great impact on the national system of rehabilitation care for that population.

The Rehabilitation Services Administration (RSA) (under the U.S. Department of Education) is the federal agency that administers and financially supports the state vocational rehabilitation agencies in each of the 50 states. This agency has recently recognized "head injury" as a unique diagnostic entity, encouraged each state agency to develop unique systems to meet the vocational needs of the brain injured, and funded several innovative demonstration projects to test new concepts in vocational rehabilitation.

The Commission for the Accreditation of Rehabilitation Facilities (CARF) is the major organization that establishes standards for rehabilitation care. Within the past several years, this agency has adopted special standards for brain injury rehabilitation that serve as a basis for accreditation of brain injury units throughout the country [40].

For many brain-injured the Disability Determination Service (DDS) is the only source of finances. Unfortunately, because the disability determination process is so heavily weighted toward physical impairments, many brain-injured patients were denied disability payments because they looked "too good." Fortunately, through the efforts of NHIF and others, the DDS has just recently revised their procedures for evaluating the brain injured; they have greatly expanded the process to include much information about cognitive and behavioral functions that may interfere with return to work. One would hope that the future will bring fairer treatment of the brain-injured claimant within the system.

CONCLUSION

Brain injury rehabilitation can be viewed from a variety of perspectives—as a scientific area of research, as a clinical program, as a "business," or as a social movement. The past decade has been rich in accomplishment: advances in research, medical practice, neuropsychological assessment, innovative treatment interventions, the mushrooming of facilities, the tremendous growth of well-trained health care professionals, increased funding, heightened public awareness, and hopefully better outcomes for our patients and families.

What challenges lie ahead? The following is a brief, and certainly not comprehensive, list of major areas in which future research and development activities should focus:

1. *More controlled studies on the relative efficacy of intensive rehabilitation programs.* As stated earlier, few studies clearly demonstrate the efficacy of rehabilitation methods in improving the outcome of brain injury. Controlled studies must be performed that clarify whether and in what manner intensive rehabilitation produces greater gains in functional abilities than either limited rehabilitation intervention or no treatment at all.

2. *Improved neurodiagnostic techniques.* The full extent of brain damage secondary to traumatic brain injury is not always apparent, even on sophisticated neurodiagnostic tests. Future developments in this field are needed to gain a better understanding of the extent of brain damage, particularly after minor brain injury.

3. *Better understanding of the process of neural recovery and methods of aiding that process.* Research currently in progress may uncover new pharmacologic and metabolic interventions that can prevent secondary cellular injury, thereby reducing morbidity and possibly decreasing mortality as well.

4. *Investigations into the effects of psychopharmacology on management of behavior problems.* Because psychopharmacologic intervention is now used more frequently as an adjunct or primary means of treating some behavioral problems, research must demonstrate which agents should be used to treat maladaptive behavior such as uncontrolled agitation, aggression, depression, and decreased initiation.

5. *Studies on the effectiveness of cognitive retraining programs.* Several studies cited above indicate that holistic cognitive remediation can improve the capacity of the brain injured to reenter the community, live independently, and return to work. Yet we do not have data that definitively indicate whether computer-assisted cognitive retraining is better than traditional cognitive rehabilitation. It is also uncertain whether cognitive therapy can improve selected cognitive functions or if the teaching of compensatory techniques is the best strategy in most cases.

6. *Better program evaluation instruments.* Program evaluation in brain injury is in its infancy. Only recently has CARF promulgated standards for evaluating acute and post-acute brain injury rehabilitation programs. Brain injury programs need to systematically use program evaluation instruments that meaningfully assess the benefits of the program for the patient and family and address the extent to which a program has improved real living skills.

7. *Development of more ecologically valid neuropsychological test procedures.* The artificiality of many neuropsychological tests limits our capacity to generalize from our test findings into real-world situations. Techniques are

sorely needed to measure everyday memory, the relationship between neuropsychological tests, the capacity to drive or to do a job, and the ability to live independently.

8. *Development of methods to sustain the effects of treatment and promote generalization.* It is unfortunate that, in some cases, the effects of intensive rehabilitation treatment are not maintained after discharge. It is incumbent on rehabilitation teams to specifically address maintenance and generalization of treatment effects. This may be accomplished by more home-based cognitive rehabilitation treatment, as well as by more systematic, long-term follow-up after a patient is discharged from the program. In certain situations, the use of "booster sessions" after a patient has been in the community for some time (e.g., 6 months) might be a good method of accomplishing this goal.

9. *Improved understanding of pediatric brain injury.* The current knowledge base of the course of recovery for infant, child, and adolescent brain injury is not as well developed as that of the adult population. Efforts should be directed toward better methods of community reentry, educational programming, and long-term management of this population.

10. *Expanded independent living and more innovative vocational rehabilitation training programs.* Only recently have independent living and vocational training programs started to include brain-injured patients in their facilities. Staff from these programs need to be trained in brain injury rehabilitation, and programs should be tailored to meet the unique neurobehavioral needs of this population, as compared with other physically disabled groups traditionally served.

11. *Better understanding of the long-term effects of minor brain injury.* Past research has led to a better understanding of the short-term sequelae of minor brain injury, namely, the postconcussion syndrome. It has also become apparent that many victims of so-called "minor" brain injury have severe cognitive and emotional problems for many months or even years after the injury.

12. *Improved use of families as therapeutic agents in the rehabilitation process.* Family treatment has become a standard part of rehabilitation practice, but the manner in which families are included in rehabilitation treatment varies greatly from program to program. There needs to be a better understanding of how and when to involve families in the rehabilitation of their relatives.

13. *More long-term residential facilities.* Many patients need extended rehabilitation, often because of persistent medical problems or severe behavior problems. Current resources appear inadequate to meet this need. In addition, a small percentage of brain-injured persons may need lifelong care. A few of these facilities have been developed recently. A needs assessment should be conducted to determine the magnitude of this problem and the projected need for such residential facilities.

A unified effort by clinicians, researchers, families and social agencies has been largely responsible for the accomplishments to date. It is imperative that research on the effectiveness of rehabilitation methods be greatly expanded. The clinician and the brain-injured victim and family must be given a basis for the belief that rehabilitation measurably and significantly affects ultimate outcome, allowing the brain-injured patient a return to social productivity and an improved quality of life.

REFERENCES

1. Glenn MB, Rosenthal M. Rehabilitation following severe traumatic brain injury. Semin Neurol 1985;5:233–46.
2. Frankowski RF, Annegers JF, Whitman S. Epidemiological and descriptive studies. Part I. The descriptive epidemiology of head trauma in the United States. In: Becker DP, Povlishock JT, eds. Central nervous system trauma status report. Richmond, VA: Byrd Press, 1985;33–43.
3. Levin HS, Kalisky Z, Handel S, Goldman AM, Eisenberg HM, Morrison D, VonLaufen A. Magnetic resonance imaging in relation to the sequelae and rehabilitation of diffuse closed head injury: Preliminary findings. Semin Neurol 1985;5:221–32.
4. Glenn MB. Anticonvulsants for prohylaxis of posttraumatic seizures. J Head Trauma Rehabil 1986;1(1):73–74.
5. Cope DN, Hall K. Head injury rehabilitation: Benefit of early intervention. Arch Phys Med Rehabil 1982;63:433–37.
6. Jennett B, Bond MR. Assessment of outcome after severe brain damage. Lancet 1975;1:480–84.
7. Rappaport M, Hall KM, Hopkins K, Belleza T. Disability rating scale for severe head trauma: Coma to community. Arch Phys Med Rehabil 1982;63:118–23.
8. Hagen C, Malkmus D, Durham P. Levels of cognitive functioning. Downey, CA: Rancho Los Amigos Professional Staff Association, 1977.
9. Levin HS, Benton AL, Grossman RG, eds. Neurobehavioral consequences of closed head injury. New York: Oxford University Press, 1982.
10. Bond MR, Brooks DN. Understanding the process of recovery as a basis for the investigation of the rehabilitation for the brain injured. Scand J Rehabil Med 1976;8:127–33.
11. Brooks N. Cognitive deficits. In: Brooks N, ed. Closed head injury: Psychological, social and family consequences. London: Oxford University Press, 1984;123–47.
12. Malkmus D. Integrating cognitive strategies into the physical therapy setting. Phys Ther 1983;63:1952–59.
13. Brooks N. Disorders of memory. In Rosenthal M, Griffith ER, Bond MR, Miller JD, eds. Rehabilitation of the head injured adult. Philadelphia: F.A. Davis, 1983;185–96.
14. Lezak M. Psychological implications of traumatic brain damage for the patient's family. Rehabil Psychol 1986;31:241–50.
15. Bond MR. Effects on the family system. In Rosenthal M, Griffith ER, Bond MR, Miller JD. Rehabilitation of the head injured adult. Philadelphia: F.A. Davis, 1983;209–18.
16. Rimel R, Giordani B, Barth J, Boll TJ, Jane JA. Disability caused by minor head injury. Neurosurgery 1981;9:221–28.
17. Hart T, Hayden M. Ecological validity of neuropsychological assessment and

remediation. In: Uzzell B, Gross Y, eds. Clinical neuropsychology of intervention. Boston, MA: Nijhoff, 1986:21–50.

18. Kay T, Silver S. The contribution of the neuropsychological evaluation to the vocational rehabilitation of the head injured adult. J Head Trauma Rehabil 1988;3(1):65–76.

19. Ben-Yishay Y, Diller L. Cognitive remediation. In: Rosenthal M, Griffith ER, Bond MR, Miller JD, eds. Rehabilitation of the head injured adult. Philadelphia: F.A. Davis, 1983:167–83.

20. Ben-Yishay Y, Rattok J, Lakin P, Piasetsky E, Ross B, Silver S, Zide E, Ezrachi O. Neuropsychologic rehabilitation: Quest for a holistic approach. Semin Neurol 1985;5:252–59.

21. Luria AR, Nayden VL, Tsvetkova LS, Vinarskaya EN. Restoration of higher brain function following brain damage. In: Vinken PJ, Bruyn GW, eds. Handbook of clinical neurology. Vol 3. Amsterdam: North Holland Publishing 1969;368–433.

22. Prigatano GP, Fordyce DJ, Zeiner HK, Rouehe JR, Peping M, Wool BC. Neuropsychological rehabilitation after closed head injury. J Neurol Neurosurg Psychiatry 1984;47:505–13.

23. Lynch WJ. The use of electronic games in cognitive rehabilitation. In: Trexler L, ed. Cognitive rehabilitation: Conceptualization and intervention. New York: Plenum Press, 1982;263–74.

24. Gianutsos R. What is cognitive rehabilitation? J Rehabil 1980;5:36–40.

25. Bracey O. Computer-based cognitive rehabilitation. Cog Rehabil 1983;1:7–8.

26. Glisky E, Schachter D. Remediation of organic memory disorders: Current status and future prospects. J Head Trauma Rehabil 1986;1(3):54–63.

27. Brooks N, Campsie L, Symington C, Beattie A, McKinlay W. The effects of severe head injury on patient and relative within seven years of injury. J Head Trauma Rehabil 1987;2(3):1–13.

28. Jacobs H, Muir C. Family training. Workshop presented at the 6th Annual National Head Injury Foundation Meeting, San Diego, CA, December 10, 1987.

29. Eames P, Wood R. Rehabilitation after severe brain injury: A follow-up study of a behavior modification approach. J Neurol Neurosurg Psychiatry 1985;48:613–19.

30. Wood RL. Behavior disorders following severe brain injury: their presentation and management. In: Brooks N, ed. Closed head injury: Psychological, social and family consequences. London: Oxford University Press, 1984;195–219.

31. Rosenbaum AH, Barry MJ. Positive therapeutic response to lithium in hypomania secondary to organic brain syndrome. Am J Psychiatry 1975;132:1072.

32. Stern J. Cranio-cerebral injured patients: A psychiatric clinical description. Scand J Rehabil Med 1978;10:7–10.

33. Mysiw WJ, Jackson RD. Tricyclic antidepressant therapy after traumatic brain injury. J Head Trauma Rehabil 1987;2(4):34–42.

34. Cope DN. Psychopharmacologic considerations in the treatment of traumatic brain injury. J. Head Trauma Rehabil 1987;2(4):1–5.

35. Helffenstein D, Wechsler F. The use of interpersonal process recall in the remediation of interpersonal and communication skill deficits in the newly brain injured. Clin Neuropsychol 1982;4:139–42.

36. Prigatano GP. Neuropsychological rehabilitation after brain injury. Baltimore: Johns Hopkins Press, 1986.

37. National Head Injury Foundation. National directory of head injury rehabilitation services. National Head Injury Foundation, Framingham, MA, 1988.

38. Mayer N, Keating D, Rapp D. Skills, routines and activity patterns of daily living: A functional nested approach. In: Uzzell B, Gross Y, eds. Clinical neuropsychology of intervention. Boston: Nijhoff, 1986;205–22.
39. Fryer LJ, Haffey WJ. Cognitive rehabilitation and community readaptation: Outcomes from two program models. J Head Trauma Rehabil 1987;2(3):51–63.
40. Commission for the Accreditation of Rehabilitation Facilities. Standards for Acute Brain Injury Rehabilitation. Tuscon, AZ, 1985.